Gynaecology

…ocus

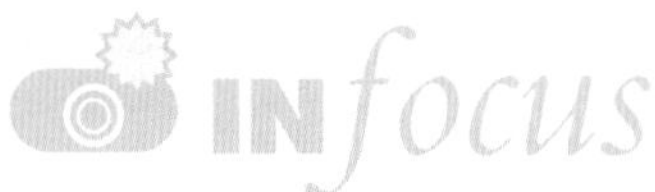

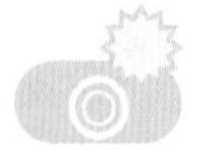

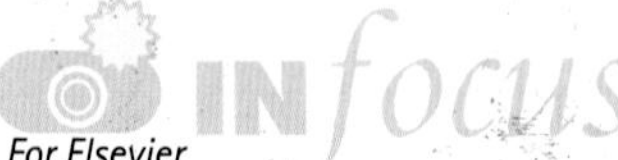

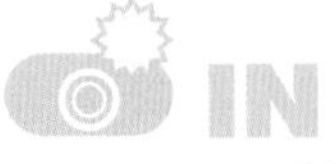

For Elsevier

Commissioning Editor: Laurence Hunter
Project Development Manager: Helen Leng
Project Manager: Frances Affleck
Design Direction: George Ajayi

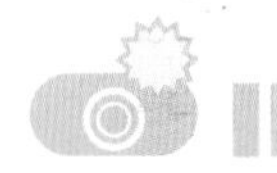

Gynaecology IN*focus*

Janice Rymer MD MRCOG FRANZCOG ILTM

Senior Lecturer/Consultant in Obstetrics and Gynaecology
Guy's, King's & St Thomas' School of Medicine
Guy's & St Thomas' Hospital Trust
London

Andrew N J Fish MD FRCOG

Consultant Gynaecologist
Brighton & Sussex University Hospitals Trust
Brighton

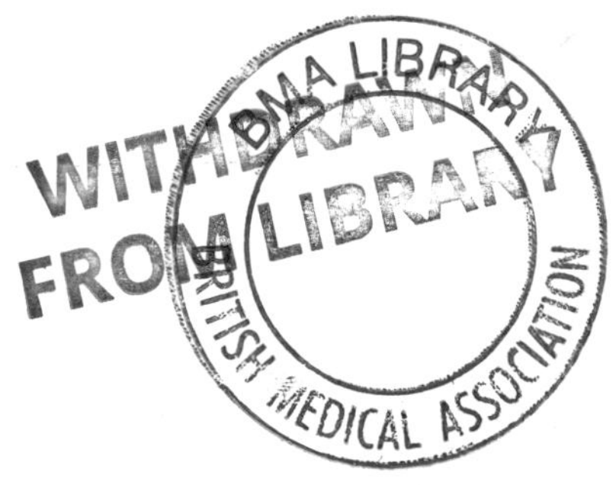

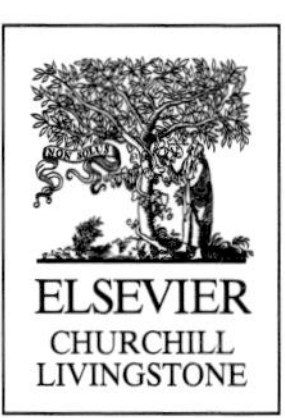

EDINBURGH LONDON NEW YORK OXFORD PHILADELPHIA ST LOUIS SYDNEY TORONTO 2005

ELSEVIER | CHURCHILL LIVINGSTONE
An imprint of Elsevier Limited

First edition 1992
Second edition 1997
Reprinted 1999
First In Focus edition 2005

[illegible]BN [illegible]0443074372

[illegible]urary Cataloguing in Publication Data
[illegible]gue record for this book is available from the British Library

[illegible]urary of Congress Cataloging in Publication Data
A [illegible]alog record for this book is available from the Library of Congress

Note

Medical knowledge is constantly changing. Standard safety precautions must be followed, but as new research and clinical experience broaden our knowledge, changes in treatment and drug therapy may become necessary or appropriate. Readers are advised to check the most current product information provided by the manufacturer of each drug to be administered to verify the recommended dose, the method and duration of administration, and contraindications. It is the responsibility of the practitioner, relying on experience and knowledge of the patient, to determine dosages and the best treatment for each individual patient. Neither the publisher nor the authors assumes any liability for any injury and/or damage to persons or property arising from this publication.

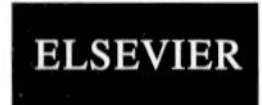

your source for books, journals and multimedia in the health sciences

www.elsevierhealth.com

The publisher's policy is to use **paper manufactured from sustainable forests**

Printed in China

Acknowledgements

We are grateful to the following for providing some of the illustrations for this book: Sir John Dewhurst, Dr R J S Harris, Dr J Robinson, Mr D H Oram, Dr S Thorpe, Dr P Greenhouse, Ms M Hooper, Dr S Barton, Dr R Jelley, Mr R Forman, Professor I Fogelman, Dr C Brown, Dr F Mitchell, Mr A Cutner, Mr C Kelleher, Mr Y Khalaf, Mrs J Robinson, Ms J Dent, Ms S Pugh, The Royal College of Surgeons, and Gower Medical Publishing. We would especially like to thank Dr E Lombardi, Mr Has Ahmed and Professor Chapman who allowed us to use material from the books that we have previously published with them. We are indebted to the photographic departments of Guy's and St Thomas' Hospital, Royal London Hospital and Brighton and Sussex University hospital, and the women who consented to being photographed.

Contents

1 Making a gynaecological diagnosis

History

A thorough history is essential to make an accurate gynaecological diagnosis.

Setting

The setting for the interview should ensure privacy and comfort for the woman, who should not be asked to undress before being interviewed.

Content

Specific information should be gathered regarding:

- parity
- last menstrual period
- length of the menstrual cycle
- contraceptive use
- date of the last cervical smear.

The presenting complaint should be clearly defined and put in the context of the previous obstetric and gynaecological history (Fig. 1). It is important to record information about sexual activity: duration of the present sexual relationship and any recent change in sexual partner. In cases of suspected infection it is mandatory to ask about the symptoms of the partner(s).

Examination: Positions

A pelvic examination can be performed with the patient either in the dorsal position or in the left lateral position (Figs 2,3). Sims position, which is similar to the coma position, may also be used. In the dorsal position the external genitalia are easily inspected, with particular reference to the vulva, labia, clitoris and urethra.

HEALTH AUTHORITY	Surname Mr Mrs Miss	Unit No.						D.O.B.		
HOSPITAL CONSULTANT	First Names									

Date	Notes	GYNAECOLOGY
	Age Parity Last Menstrual Period –/–/–	
	Cycle / Contraception Last Cervical Smear –/–/–	
	Presenting Problem	
	Previous Obstetric and Gynaecological History	
	Previous Medical History	
	Social History / Family History Drugs	
	Allergies	
	Clinical Findings	

Fig. 1 History sheet.

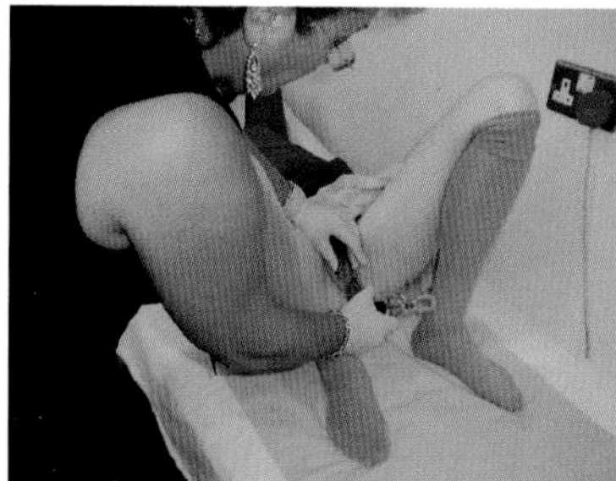

Fig. 2 Examination in the dorsal position.

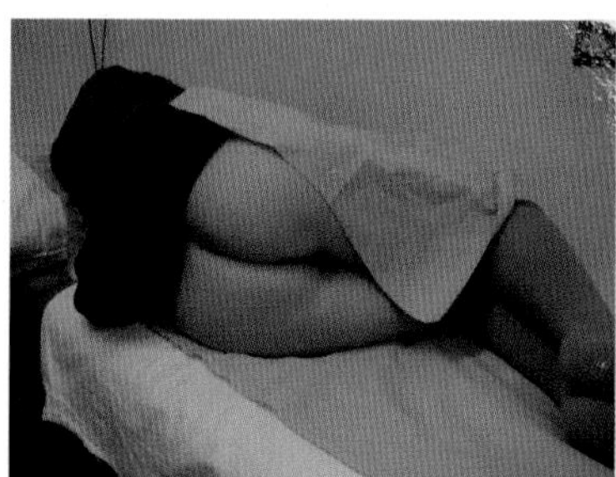

Fig. 3 Patient in the left lateral position.

Examination: Instruments and techniques

Bivalve speculum

A bivalve speculum is used to inspect the cervix and the vaginal walls (Fig. 4). It is also used when taking cervical smears and endocervical swabs.

Bimanual examination

A bimanual examination is performed to assess the pelvic organs. Gloves are used on both hands. One or two lubricated fingers of the right hand are inserted into the vagina and used to elevate and steady the uterus and adnexa so that the left hand on the abdomen can feel the pelvic organs (Fig. 5). The size, position (anteverted, axial or retroverted) and mobility of the uterus are determined together with the presence of tenderness and/or masses in the fornices. *Cervical excitation* is defined as tenderness that arises in one or other adnexum when the broad ligament is stretched by movement of the cervix with the examining fingers.

Sims speculum

The left lateral position facilitates the use of a Sims speculum (Fig. 6). This instrument was originally designed for displaying vesicovaginal fistulae. It is now more often used in the assessment of uterovaginal prolapse. One end of the speculum is inserted into the vagina and gentle traction is applied backwards. The anterior vaginal wall is thus visualized. To view the posterior vaginal wall, a pair of sponge-holding forceps are inserted to retract the anterior vaginal wall while the Sims speculum is slowly withdrawn.

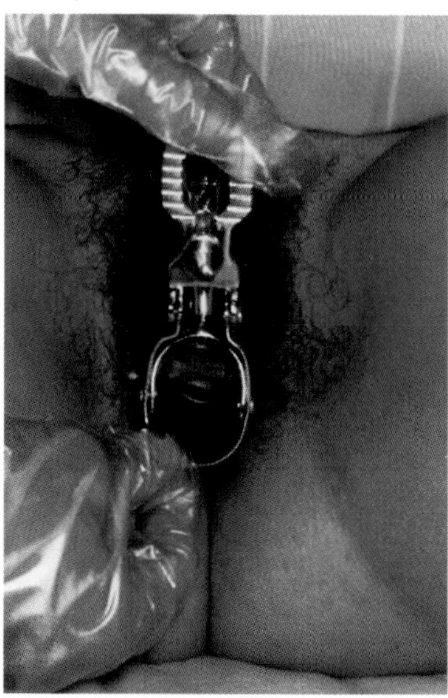

Fig. 4 Examination with a bivalve speculum.

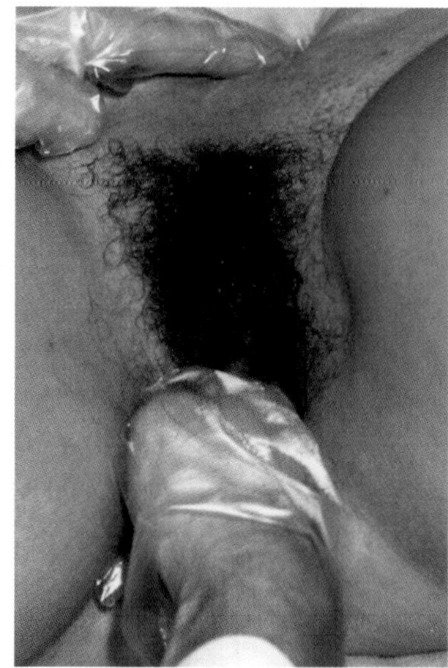

Fig. 5 Bimanual examination.

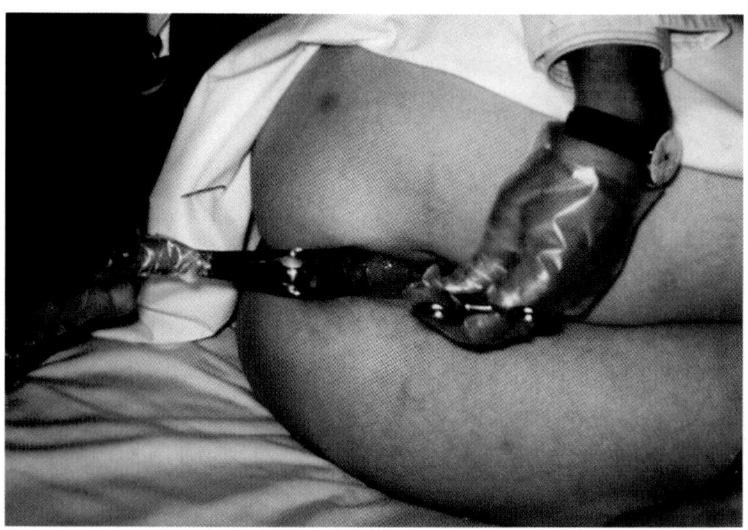

Fig. 6 Examination using a Sims speculum.

2 Investigative techniques

Taking a cervical smear

The cervix should be clearly visualized using a bivalve speculum. The narrow point of the wooden spatula is inserted into the endocervical canal so that the lip rests against the cervix (Fig. 7). It is then rotated through 360°, keeping in firm contact with the cervix, and then removed. The material collected on the spatula is spread evenly on a microscope slide (Fig. 8a) which is immediately immersed in fixative (3% acetic acid in 95% alcohol).

Liquid-based cytology is being introduced. The sample is taken as in Figure 7 and agitated in the transport medium (Fig. 8b) enabling the laboratory to prepare slides that are easier to read.

Indications

All sexually active women should have smears taken at 3-yearly intervals. The National Cervical Screening Programme in the UK includes all women 20–65 years, 3–5-yearly.

Taking microbiological swabs

High vaginal swabs are taken from the posterior fornix using a bivalve speculum. The cotton-tipped swab is placed in the appropriate transport medium.

Indications

High vaginal swabs are used to detect lower genital tract pathogens, e.g. *Candida albicans* or *Trichomonas vaginalis*, which give rise to symptoms such as discharge and vulval irritation. Endocervical swabs are used to detect pathogens that may spread to the upper genital tract and cause pelvic inflammatory disease, e.g. *Chlamydia trachomatis* and *Neisseria gonorrhoeae*. These bacteria infect columnar epithelium. The microbiological swab should be inserted into the endocervical canal (Fig. 9), agitated and withdrawn. It should then be placed in the appropriate transport medium.

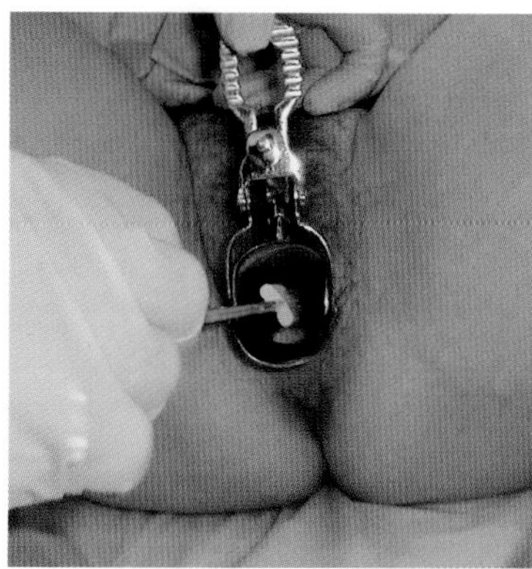

Fig. 7 Taking a cervical smear.

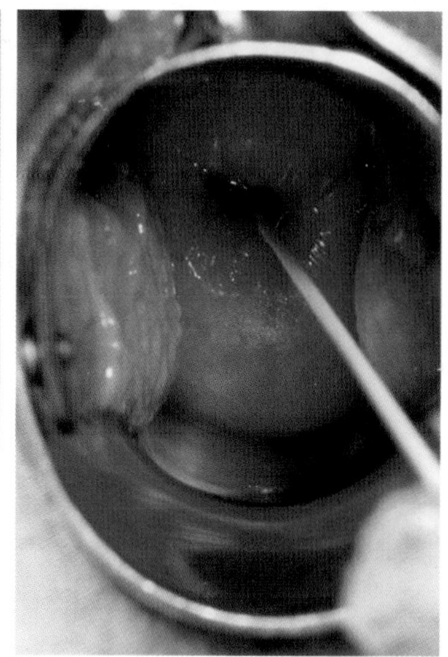

Fig. 9 Taking an endocervical swab.

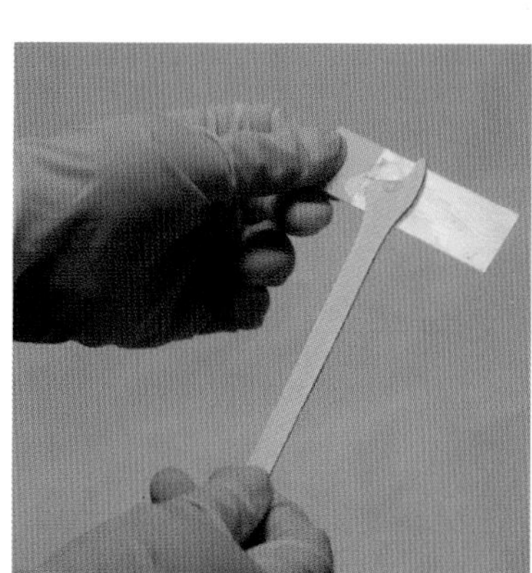

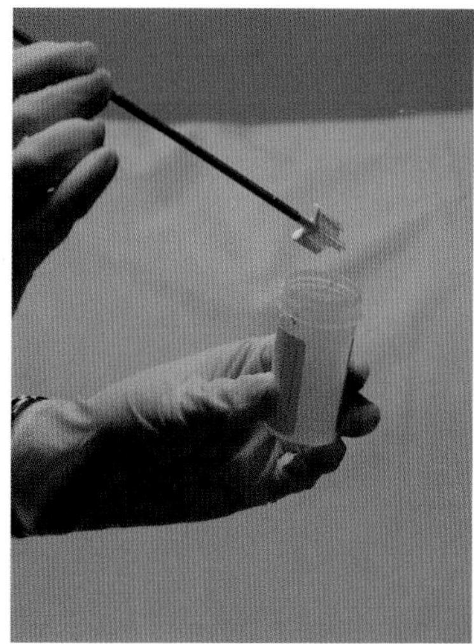

Fig. 8 a. Spreading the smear on a microscope slide. b. Specimen for liquid based cytology.

Colposcopy

Indications

All women who have had cervical smears showing borderline changes or mild dyskaryosis that does not resolve spontaneously, or those women with a single smear showing moderately or severely dyskaryotic cells, should be referred for colposcopy.

Description

The colposcope (Fig. 10) is a binocular microscope. An illuminated, three-dimensional view of the cervix is obtained, magnified between 6 and 40 times (Fig. 11). This technique identifies both the severity of the abnormality giving rise to an abnormal smear and also its position on the cervix. Hence it allows the clinician to assess the suitability for local ablative therapy.

Technique

The patient is examined in the lithotomy position and a bivalve speculum is used to expose the cervix. Cotton wool swabs are then used to clean mucus off the cervix before applying 5% acetic acid to stain the abnormal areas white (acetowhite). If the upper limit of the transformation zone lies within the endocervical canal, forceps may be useful in exposing the whole area (Fig. 12). If the upper limit of the transformation zone cannot be visualized then the examination must be considered incomplete. This occurs in less than 10% of women aged 25 years or less, but in more than 30% of women over the age of 40 years.

Punch biopsy forceps can be used to obtain a sample from colposcopically abnormal areas to make a histological diagnosis. Once the results of this are known, ablative treatment such as Semm cautery or laser can be applied. Diathermy loop excision (DLE) of the transformation zone is used to excise cervical lesions. For women with moderate or severely dyskaryotic smears and colposcopic changes consistent with this, the treatment process removes the abnormality and produces a good sample for histological analysis, thus enabling assessment and treatment at one visit (see and treat).

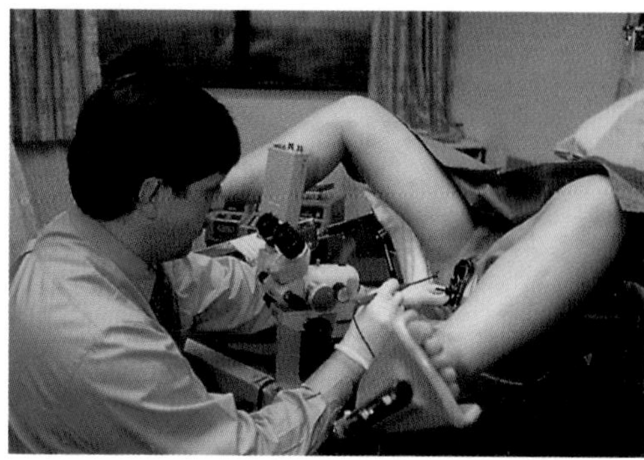

Fig. 10 Colposcopy clinic.

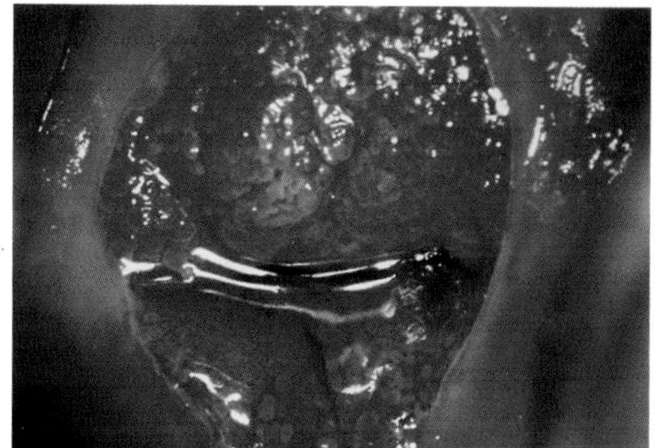

Fig. 11 Colpophotograph of a normal cervix.

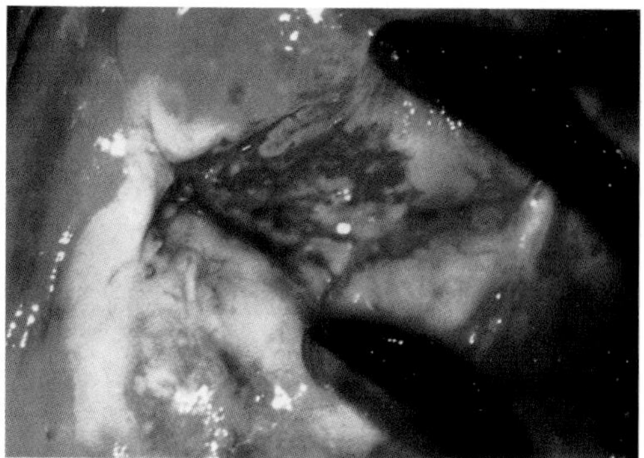

Fig. 12 Exposing the squamocolumnar junction.

Ultrasound

Description

Ultrasonography records high-frequency sound waves as they are reflected from anatomic structures. Ultrasound waves are mechanical waves beyond the scope of hearing. When they are directed toward media of differing densities, the sound waves spread out with differing velocities. Echoes arise at the interfaces between these media, and the greater the density differences the greater the intensity of the echoes. This echo signal is measured and converted into a clinical picture of the area under examination. Thus, for good visualization there must be an air-free coupling of the transducer to the abdomen. Ultrasound is a simple and painless procedure that has no known ill-effects. The ultrasonographer and patient can look at the ultrasound image together (Fig. 13).

Various probes are now available (Fig. 14). If an abdominal probe is used, the scan is performed with a full bladder which provides a sonographic 'window'. A vaginal probe eliminates the need to have a full bladder, which is especially useful in early pregnancy.

Indications

Ultrasonography is useful in almost any pelvic abnormality as all structures can usually be demonstrated either by transvaginal or abdominal scanning. Blood flow to various organs can be demonstrated using Colour Doppler techniques (Fig. 15).

The first sign of an intrauterine pregnancy can be detected in the 5th week as a small, sharply outlined cavity which is the gestational sac. Between the 7th and 8th weeks, embryonic structures can be visualized as distinct echoes. The fetal heart can be seen beating from 5 weeks if a transvaginal probe is used.

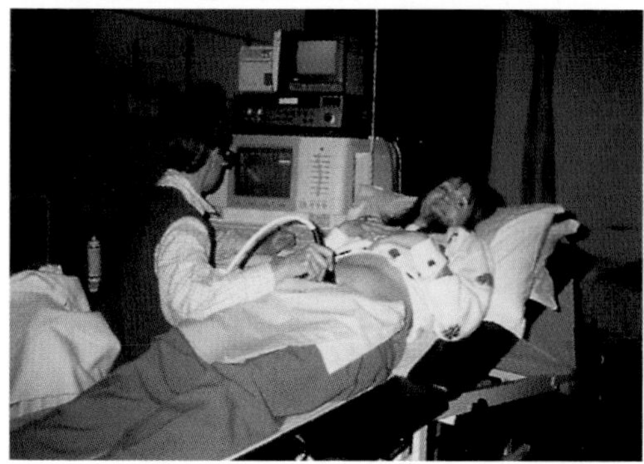

Fig. 13 An abdominal ultrasound being performed.

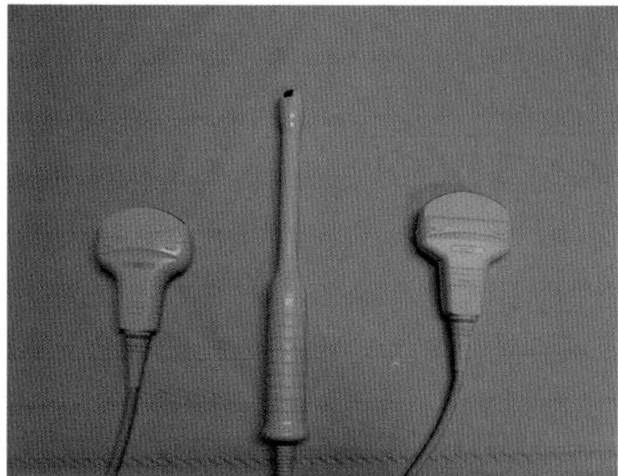

Fig. 14 Vaginal and abdominal ultrasound probes.

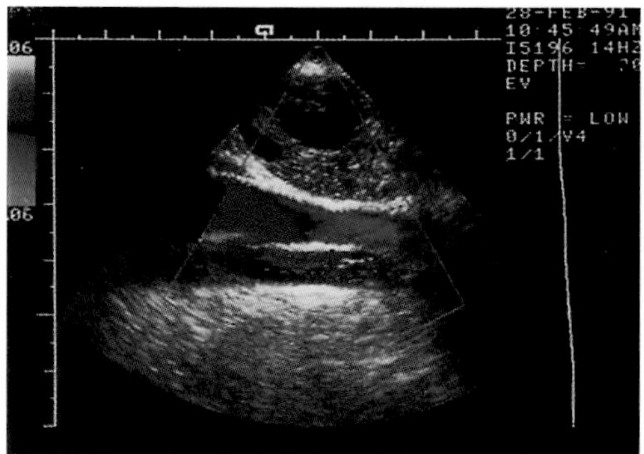

Fig. 15 Colour Doppler ultrasound illustrating normal ovarian blood flow.

Hysterosalpingography

Description

Hysterosalpingography (HSG) is an X-ray method of assessing fallopian tube patency and demonstrating structural abnormalities of the uterine cavity.

Indications

HSG will show whether the fallopian tubes are patent. If not, the area in which the tubes are blocked can be identified. It will not give information concerning the condition of the pelvis, i.e. the presence of peritubular adhesions and/or pelvic distortion which may impair fertility even though the tubes are patent.

Technique

HSG is usually performed without anaesthetic in the X-ray department. A bivalve speculum is used to expose the cervix which is cannulated to enable radiopaque dye to be injected into the uterine cavity. The procedure is viewed using an image intensifier and recorded on film (Fig. 16).

HyCoSy (hysterosalpingo contrast sonography)

An alternative technique to assess tubal patency whereby an echogenic suspension is inserted into the uterine cavity, which then flows through the tubes under ultrasonic surveillance (Fig. 17).

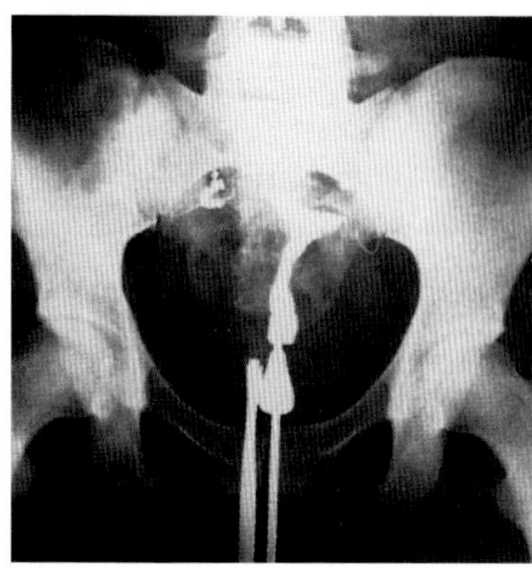

Fig. 16 Hysterosalpingogram outlining the uterine and tubal anatomy.

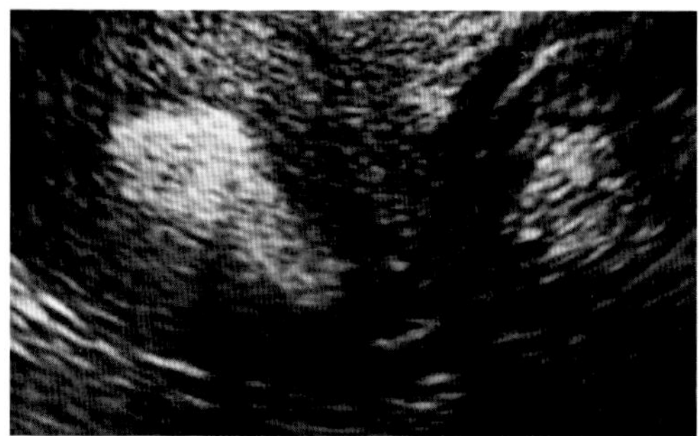

Fig. 17 Hysterosalpingo contrast sonography (HyCoSy).

Hysteroscopy

Description and technique

Hysteroscopy is a method that enables visual examination of the uterine cavity. A hysteroscope is a telescope surrounded by a sheath. It is inserted into the uterine cavity through the cervix with the patient in the lithotomy position and under either local or general anaesthesia.

Indications

Endometrial polyps, fibroids and adhesions within the uterine cavity can be visualized hysteroscopically, together with different types of endometrium, e.g. normal, hyperplastic, atrophic and malignant (Figs 18–20). It is also possible to use the hysteroscope to take endometrial biopsies, divide adhesions, and remove polyps and misplaced IUCDs. The endometrial lining can be removed using an electrical resection loop or laser in women with menorrhagia. Submucous fibroids can also be removed in this way.

Complications

Complications of the procedure include perforation of the uterus, infection and fluid overload (e.g. if fluid distension medium is used for endometrial resection).

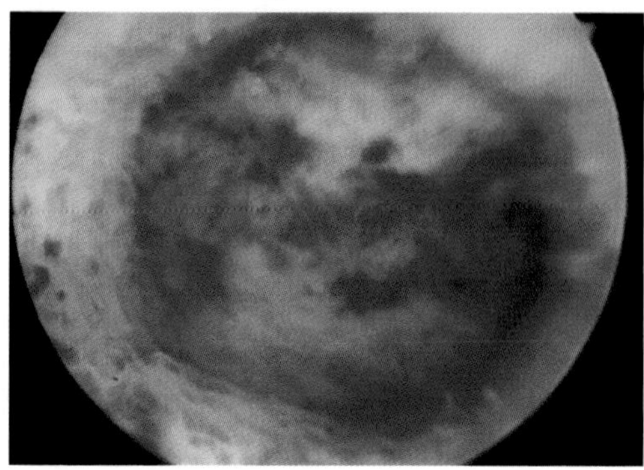

Fig. 18 Normal endometrium.

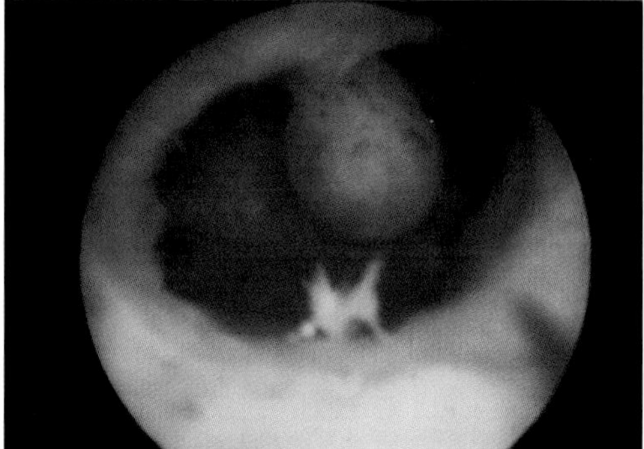

Fig. 19 Endometrial polyp.

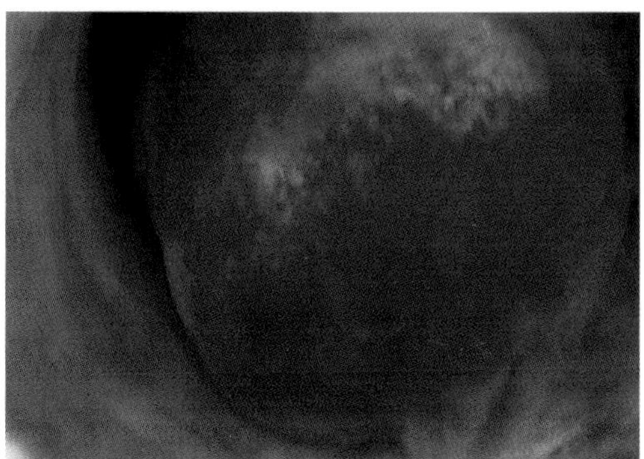

Fig. 20 Endometrial pedunculated fibroid.

Laparoscopy

Description

The laparoscope is essentially a telescope that is inserted into the abdominal cavity after it has been inflated with carbon-dioxide. The direct view obtained allows the diagnosis of gynaecological disorders and surgery (Figs 21, 22) without laparotomy.

Technique

The procedure is almost invariably performed under general anaesthesia with the patient paralysed and ventilated. The patient is placed in the modified Lloyd–Davies position with the head down. The bladder is catheterized. A small incision is made at the umbilicus and a Veress needle is inserted into the peritoneal cavity. Carbon dioxide is insufflated into the peritoneal cavity to a pressure of 20 mmHg. The needle is withdrawn and the laparoscopic trocar and cannula are inserted. The trocar is withdrawn and replaced with the laparoscope, which allows direct visualization of the pelvic organs (Fig. 23). If needed, further cannulae are inserted under direct laparoscopic vision, suprapubically or in either iliac fossa, to permit manipulation of pelvic organs and instrumentation for various surgical techniques.

Indications

These include pelvic pain, diagnosis and treatment of ectopic pregnancy, infertility investigation, sterilization, trauma, lost IUCD and assisted conception techniques, as well as staging procedures for gynaecological cancer, including pelvic lymph node sampling. More advanced procedures include laparoscopically assisted vaginal hysterectomy (LAVH), laparoscopic colposuspension and laparoscopic sacrocolpopexy.

Complications

Complications of the procedure include:

- Pain, especially shoulder-tip pain from CO_2 diaphragmatic irritation
- Bleeding
- Puncture of bladder, bowel
- Misplacement of gas
- Mortality rate approximately 1 in 15,000.

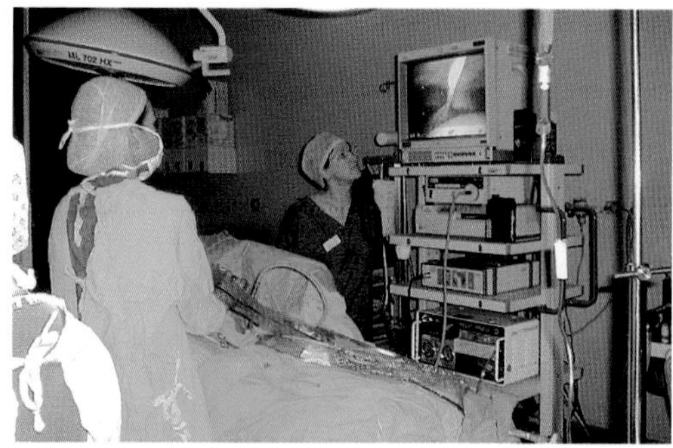

Fig. 21 Laparoscopy being performed.

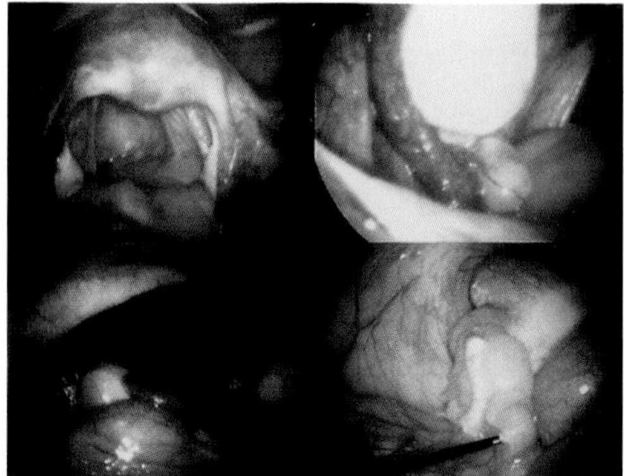

Fig. 22 Laparoscopic views of internal organs.

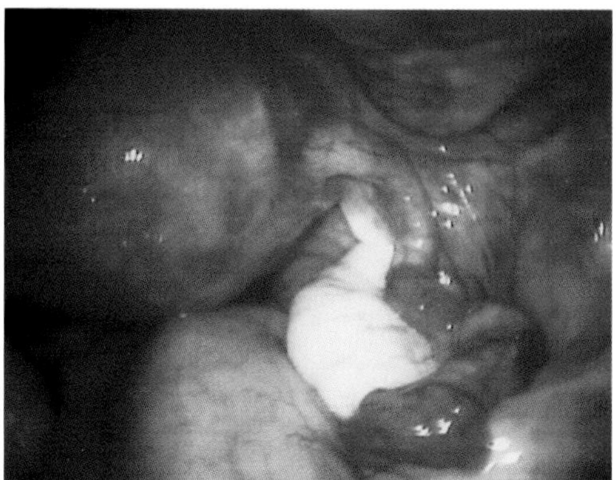

Fig. 23 Normal fallopian tube and ovary as seen with laparoscopy.

3 Childhood gynaecological disorders

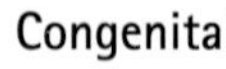

Congenital

Hydrocolpos

In this disorder, an imperforate membrane is situated immediately above the hymen. Above this obstruction the vagina can become distended by fluid (Fig. 24). Hydrocolpos can present in the neonate as retention of urine, abdominal pain and a lower abdominal swelling if there is a large quantity of fluid. The treatment is simple incision of the membrane to release the fluid.

Haematocolpos

The same situation as in hydrocolpos occurs in haematocolpos, except that the problem does not arise until puberty. The menstrual fluid is unable to be released and collects above the imperforate hymen, grossly expanding the vagina and even the uterus. The presenting symptoms may include abdominal pain, urinary retention or a large abdominal mass. Vulval inspection will reveal a bulging bluish membrane that requires incision.

Fused labia

The labia minora become adherent to each other (Fig. 25), and it may appear as though the vagina is absent. The aetiology is not known, but the condition is probably due to low oestrogen levels. Application of oestrogen cream usually results in spontaneous separation after 10–14 days.

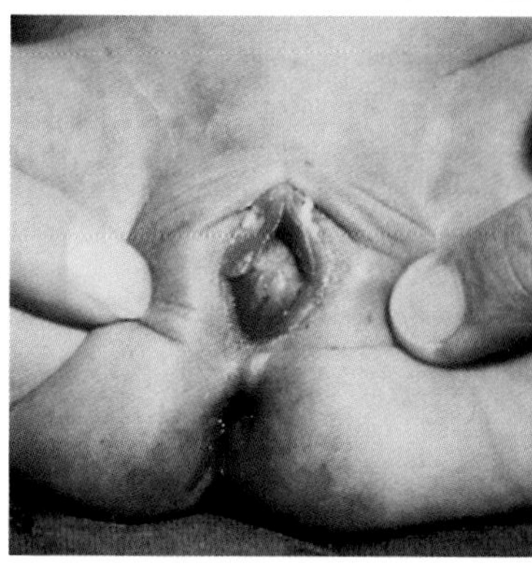

Fig. 24 Hydrocolpos.

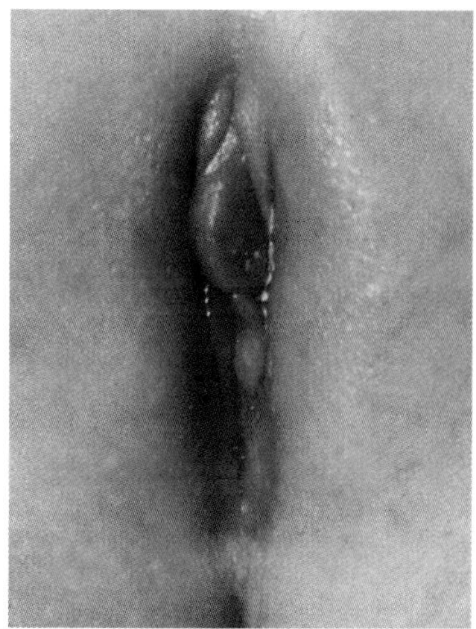

Fig. 25 Fused labia.

Congenital abnormalities

The müllerian ducts are the embryological precursors of the fallopian tubes, uterus and upper two-thirds of the vagina. The lower one-third of the vagina develops from the urogenital sinus. Various defects can occur during embryological development (Fig. 26). These include failure of:

- development, e.g. no paramesonephric duct
- paramesonephric duct canalization
- fusion of paramesonephric ducts
- median septum loss (Fig. 27)
- fundal dome development
- fusion of paramesonephric ducts with urogenital sinus
- transverse septum loss between paramesonephric system and urogenital sinus.

Problems in early childhood

Vulvovaginitis

This is the most common gynaecological problem in children. There are three factors that make the immature vagina susceptible to infection:

- lack of protective acid secretion
- contamination by stool and debris
- impaired mechanisms of immunity.

The usual bacteriological finding is of mixed bacterial flora. The child will complain of vulval soreness, discharge, or pain on micturition. Threadworm infestation can sometimes cause this condition.

Foreign bodies

These usually produce a purulent discharge or bleeding.

Botryoid sarcoma

Tumours are rare in childhood but embryonal rhabdomyosarcoma is the most serious. It is often grapelike in appearance (Fig. 28) but may appear simply as a polyp. The tumour spreads extensively in the subepithelial tissues of the vagina or ectocervix. Chemotherapy is generally given prior to extended hysterectomy or vaginectomy (Fig. 29).

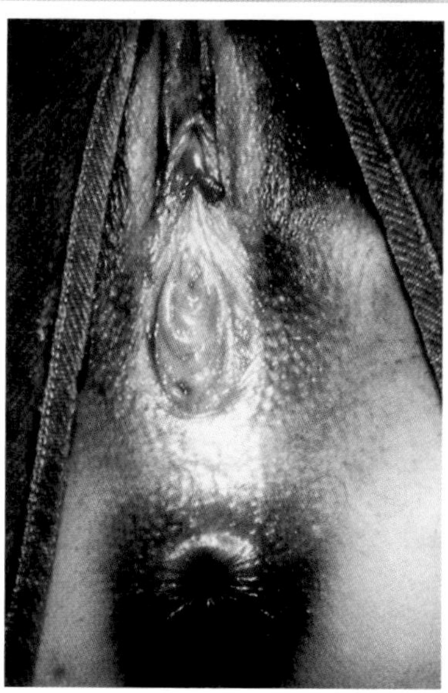

Fig. 26 Absent vagina – a congenital defect.

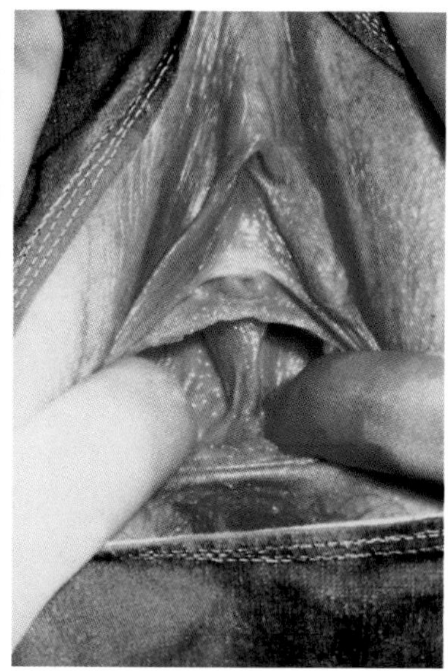

Fig. 27 Vaginal septum.

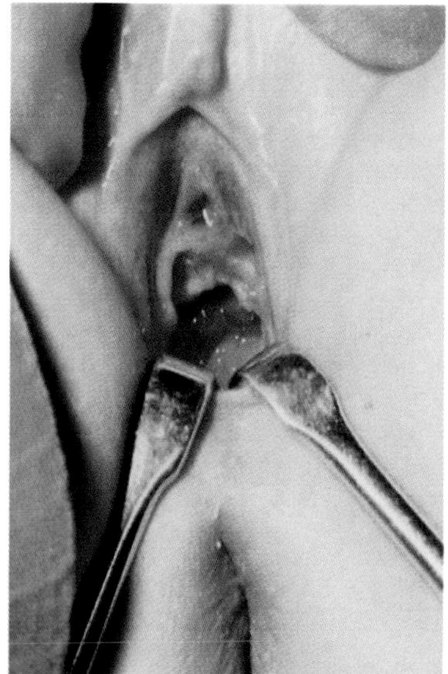

Fig. 28 Botryoid sarcoma at examination.

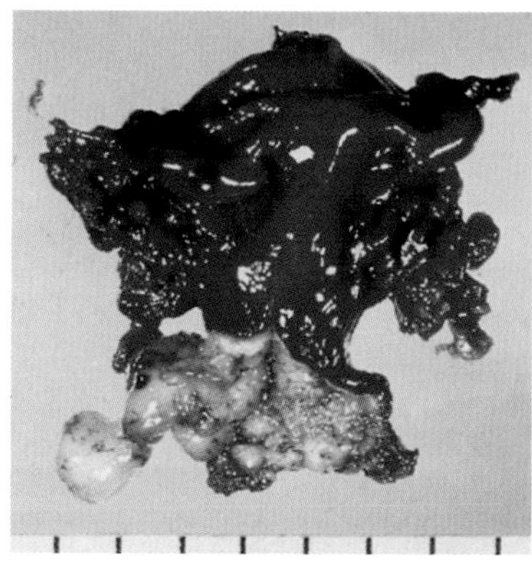

Fig. 29 Surgical specimen of botryoid sarcoma.

Sexual abuse

Children who have been sexually abused endure physical and psychological trauma. When sexual abuse is suspected, a thorough examination must be carried out by an experienced gynaecologist. Swabs for sexually transmitted diseases must be taken from the vagina, cervix and anus. Samples for semen should also be taken. Photographs should be taken if possible, and the signs of physical trauma should be accurately documented. The examinations are often performed under anaesthesia.

Vulval bruising is common, and the hymen is often perforated (Fig. 30). Anal bruising must be looked for (Fig. 31), and anal dilatation. The rest of the body must be searched for bruising or other signs of trauma. Fractures should be suspected. These children usually need to be admitted until the domestic situation has been thoroughly investigated. A multidisciplinary approach involving social workers, paediatricians and gynaecologists is usually adopted.

Female genital mutilation

This custom is still practised, mainly in Africa. It is illegal in the UK. The extent of the procedure varies from trimming of the labia minora to complete removal of the labia and clitoris with sewing over of the vaginal introitus. Complications are common. If the operation is carried out near puberty, haemorrhage and sepsis can be severe. When complete excision of the labia and minora is performed, the denuded edges are encouraged to unite by strapping the thighs together, with a stick between the edges to allow passage of urine. The resulting scarring can be extreme and the urethra and vestibule hidden (Fig. 32). Epidermoid cysts can result (Fig. 33). This deflects the urinary stream causing chronic infection both of the surrounding skin and vagina. Intercourse may be impossible, and division of a skin bridge may be necessary. For vaginal delivery, an anterior episiotomy may be necessary. In obstructed labour, the fetus may be in the vagina for long enough to cause vaginal wall pressure necrosis.

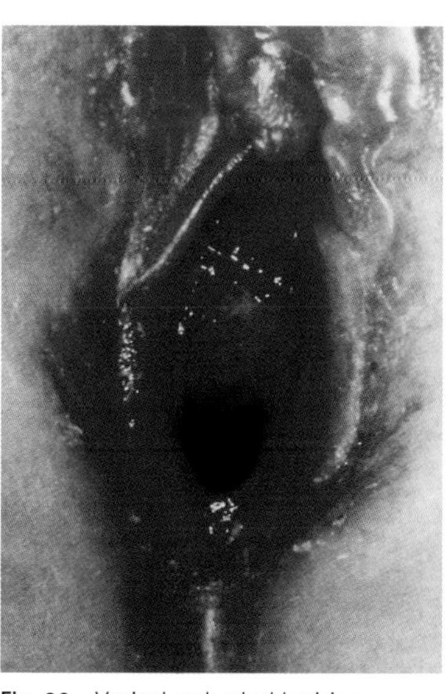

Fig. 30 Vaginal and vulval bruising.

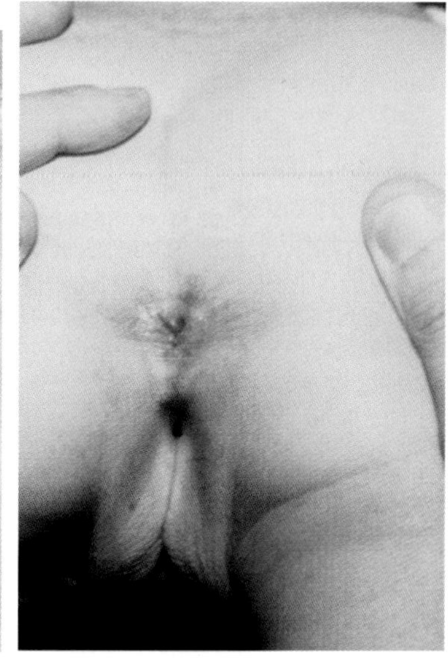

Fig. 31 Anal trauma.

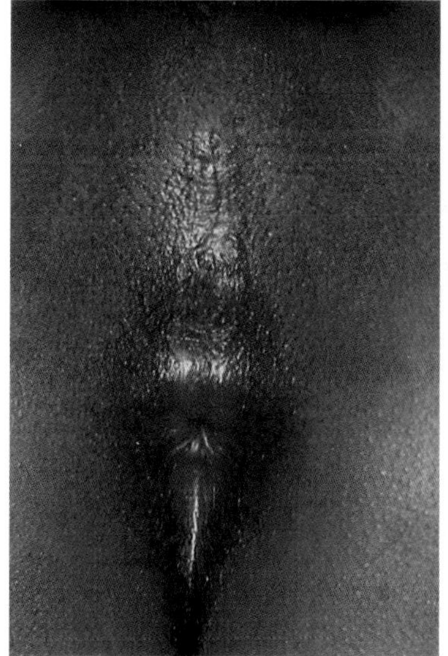

Fig. 32 Female genital mutilation.

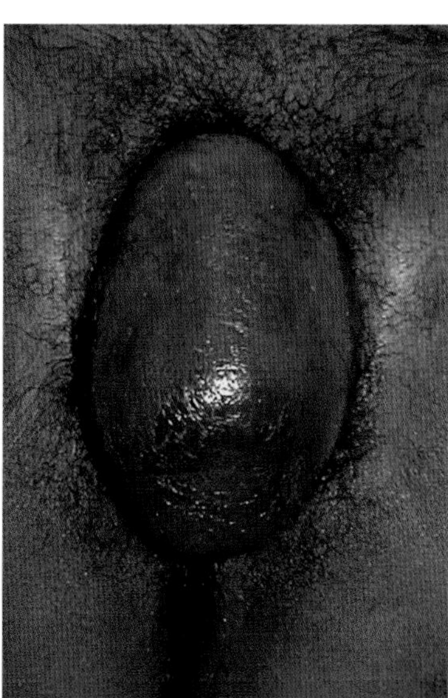

Fig. 33 An epidermoid cyst as a result of female genital mutilation.

Disorders of puberty

The hormonal changes of puberty are complex. Disordered function can reveal chromosomal, enzymatic and structural abnormalities not obvious in childhood.

Turner's syndrome

In Turner's syndrome (Fig. 34), the absence of the one sex chromosome leads to ovarian dysgenesis resulting in primary amenorrhoea, short stature and sexual infantilism. Alternatively, androgen-receptor defects with a normal XY complement lead to failure of masculinization and apparently normal, full breast development. Primary amenorrhoea may be the first presentation of testicular feminization (Fig. 35).

5α reductase deficiency

In 5α reductase deficiency (Fig. 36), the lack of the enzyme likewise results in failure of masculinization of the external genitalia in the genotypic male child. However, at puberty the large increase in testosterone production by normal, internalized testes results in androgenization of the presumed female. The testes are removed and oestrogen replacement ensures a phenotypic female.

Other problems include precocious puberty, as indicated by early thelarche or menarche, or delayed puberty where hypothalamic maturation is pathologically late.

Intersex

Definition

An intersex is an individual in whom there is discordance between chromosomal, gonadal, internal genital and phenotype sex, or the sex of rearing.

Clinical features

It may be declared at birth because of ambiguous external genitalia (Fig. 37), during childhood because of precocious puberty or during adolescence because pubertal changes are inappropriate to presumed gender, or because puberty fails to occur.

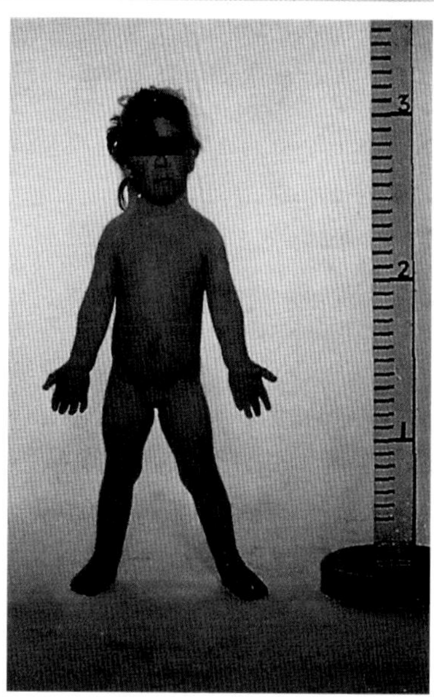

Fig. 34 Turner's syndrome.

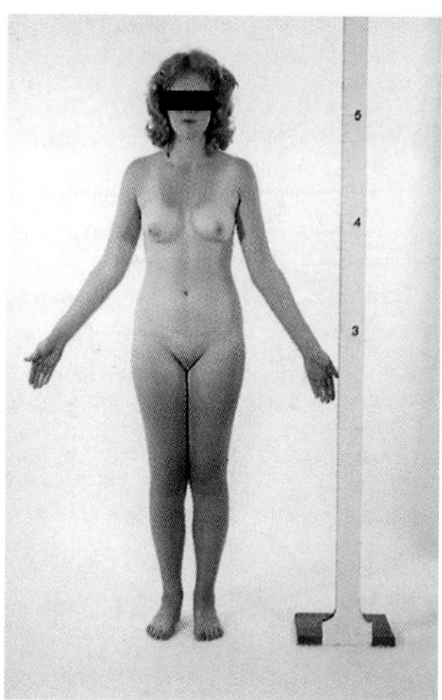

Fig. 35 Testicular feminization.

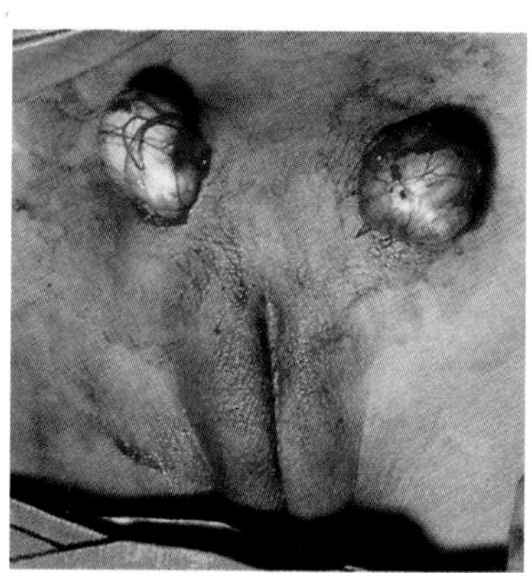

Fig. 36 Inguinal testes in 5α reductase deficiency.

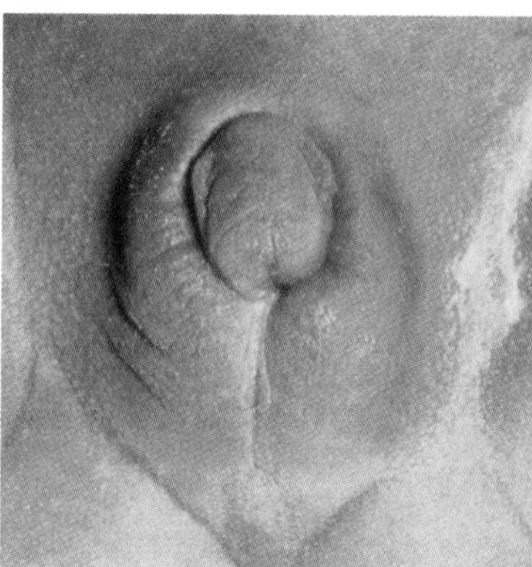

Fig. 37 Intersex.

4 The menstrual cycle

Puberty

At puberty the HPO axis changes and GnRH is secreted in a pulsatile fashion from the hypothalamus. This stimulates a pulsatile release of FSH and LH from the anterior pituitary. Thereafter, FSH and LH are secreted in pulses every 70–220 min depending on the cycle phase. The release of the gonadotrophins is regulated by the ovarian steroid feedback on the hypothalamus and pituitary.

Hormonal changes

At the beginning of each cycle (Fig. 38a), FSH stimulates growth in follicles, with one follicle becoming dominant while the others undergo atresia. Oestrogen production in the dominant follicle increases, leading to rising estradiol blood levels, which trigger the LH surge from the pituitary, in turn causing ovulation. This LH surge also stimulates the production of progesterone and prostaglandins in the follicle. The oocyte is then released from the follicle, which shrinks and becomes the progesterone-producing corpus luteum. Unless a pregnancy occurs, this regresses after about 10 days. If pregnancy occurs, the HCG maintains the production of steroids from the corpus luteum until week 10 of pregnancy.

Endometrial changes

The endometrium in the first half of the cycle (Fig. 38b) responds to the oestrogenic stimulation by growth of the glands and endometrial thickening. When progesterone is produced in the second half of the cycle, the epithelium lining the glands develops vacuoles, and the glands and the spiral arterioles continue to grow. The stroma becomes oedematous and undergoes decidualization.

Falling levels of oestrogen and progesterone cause cyclical constriction and dilatation of the spiral arterioles; eventually generalized vasoconstriction, ischaemia and cell disintegration occur leading to release of lysosomal enzymes. Breakdown is halted by rising levels of oestrogen from the next follicle. The cervix and vagina show changes in response to ovarian steroid output (Fig. 39).

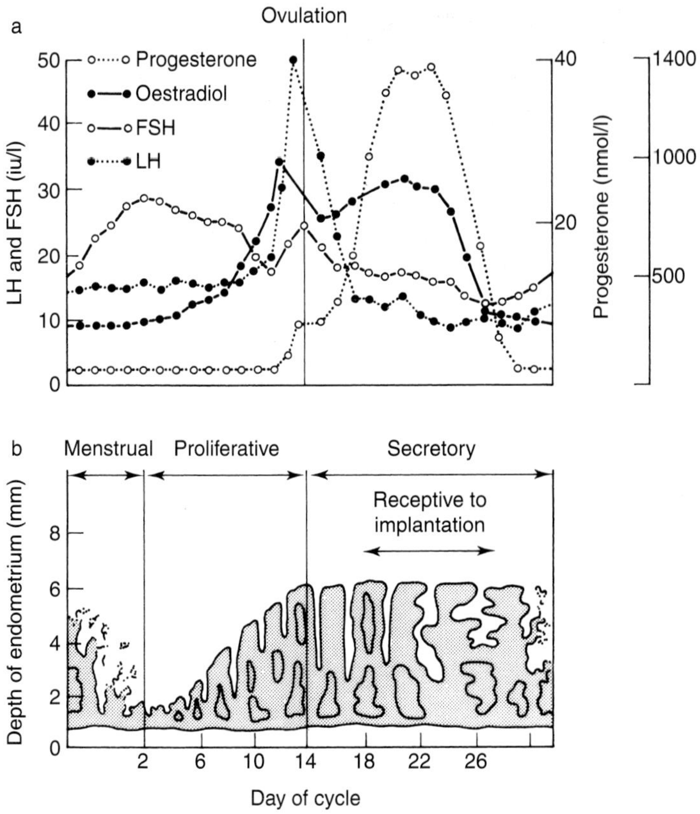

Fig. 38 The menstrual cycle. (a) Hormonal changes. (b) Endometrial changes.

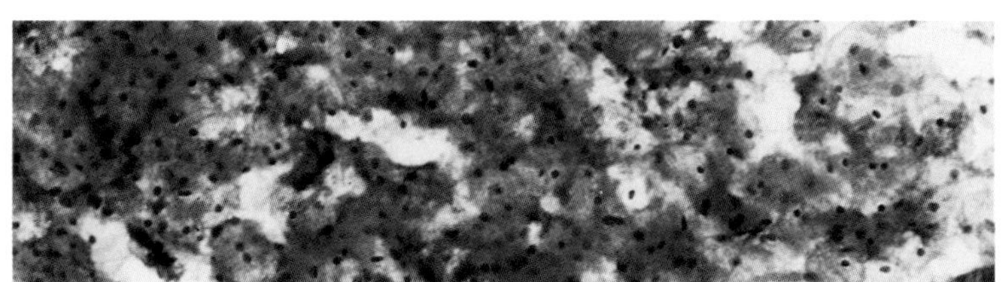

Fig. 39 Vaginal cytology showing oestrogenic stimulation.

Amenorrhoea

Amenorrhoea is defined as the failure to menstruate. It can be classified as primary (menstruation fails to start) or secondary, which is defined as the cessation of periods for more than 6 months. Amenorrhoea may be due to the absence of the uterus, as in an XY female, blockage of the outflow tract owing to an imperforate hymen, or endometrial disturbances, i.e. absence as in uterine scarring (Asherman syndrome), atrophy as in premature menopause, or hormonal imbalance as in polycystic ovarian syndrome.

Primary

Primary amenorrhoea has been mentioned in disorders of puberty (pg. 24).

Secondary

The most common causes of secondary amenorrhoea are hypothalamic suppression (Fig. 40), hyperprolactinaemia (usually due to a prolactinoma, Fig. 41) or polycystic ovarian syndrome. Other causes include thyroid disease, adrenal disease, premature ovarian failure and Sheehan syndrome. Sheehan syndrome is a form of hypopituitarism caused by post-partum ischaemic necrosis of the anterior pituitary. The hyperplastic pituitary gland in pregnancy is more susceptible to hypotension and severe post-partum haemorrhage may precipitate Sheehan syndrome.

Asherman syndrome should be suspected in women who have amenorrhoea and have normal hormonal profiles with evidence of ovulation, particularly in women who have had some form of uterine surgery, for example termination of pregnancy or dilatation and curettage (D&C), which could precipitate the formation of intrauterine adhesions. Pregnancy and natural menopause are physiological courses of amenorrhoea. When a woman presents with secondary amenorrhea pregnancy and natural menopause should always be considered.

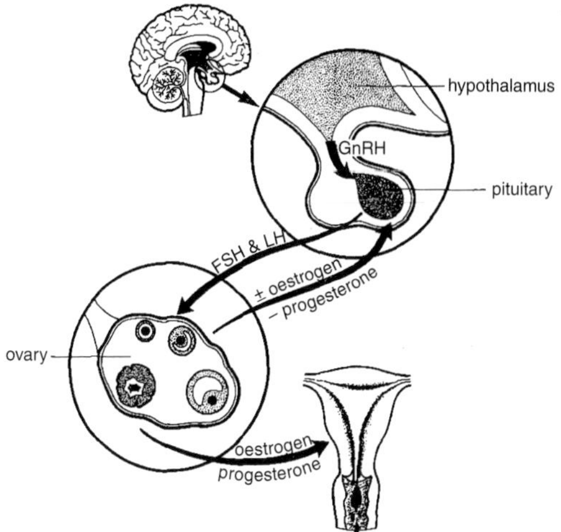

Fig. 40 Hypothalamic–pituitary–ovarian axis.

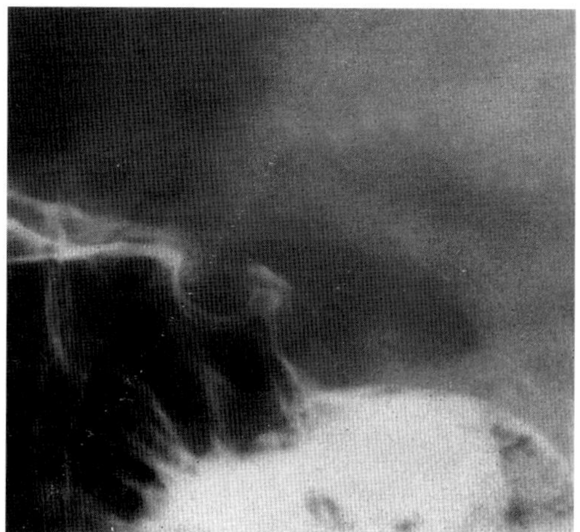

Fig. 41 Skull X-ray of enlarged pituitary fossa.

Dysfunctional uterine bleeding

Definition

Abnormal uterine bleeding after pelvic pathology has been excluded.

Aetiology

Not known.

Classification

Cases can be divided into anovulatory or ovulatory.

Clinical features

The majority of patients will report heavy bleeding, which may be regular or irregular. It is extremely difficult to make an accurate assessment of the amount of bleeding by relying on history alone. Quantitative measurement of blood loss can be made by collecting all the tampons and sanitary pads and using the alkalin haematin test but is rarely done in clinical practice.

On abdominal and pelvic examination there should be no abnormalities detected.

Investigations

To exclude pelvic pathology, a thorough pelvic assessment must be made including cervical smear, transvaginal ultrasound (Fig. 42), and endometrial biopsy (Fig. 43) if indicated. Laparoscopy, hysteroscopy (Fig. 44) or colour Doppler studies may be used, depending on the clinical situation.

Management

Anovulatory In adolescents the oral contraceptive pill will make the withdrawal bleeds lighter, regular and less painful. In the perimenopausal woman, hormone replacement therapy or cyclical progestogens (after exclusion of uterine pathology) would be appropriate.

Ovulatory Non-steroidal anti-inflammatory drugs, the oral contraceptive pill, danazol and antifibrinolytic drugs or the progesterone-releasing intrauterine system (IUS) are the main options. Endometrial resection/ablation or hysterectomy are used if the above measures fail.

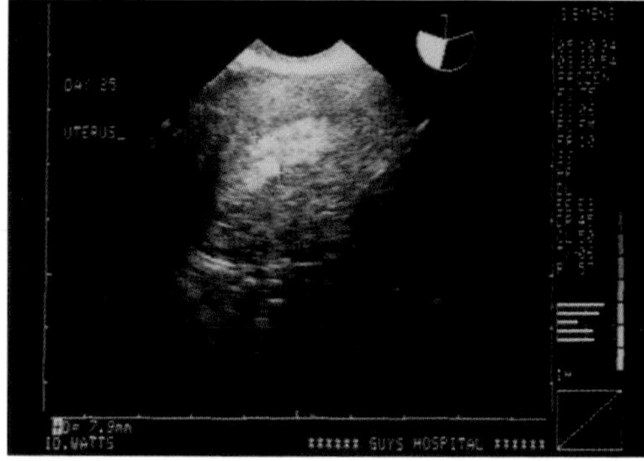

Fig. 42 Transvaginal ultrasound scan of endometrium.

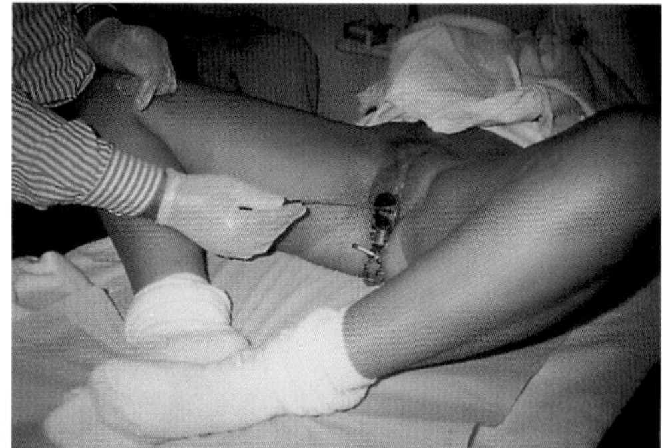
Fig. 43 Endometrial biopsy.

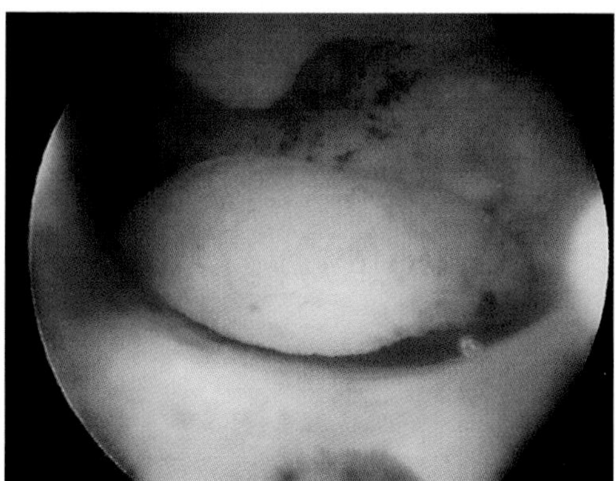
Fig. 44 Hysteroscopic view of an endometrial polyp.

5 Contraception

'Natural' methods

Highest fertility occurs at ovulation: in a 28-day cycle this occurs about 14 days after the last menstrual period. Sperm may survive in the genital tract for up to 7 days; therefore, to avoid conception, discontinue intercourse one week before ovulation is expected and recommence it not less than 2 days after ovulation has occurred. Ovulation may be predicted by:

- monitoring previous cycles (rhythm method)
- using the rise in body temperature with ovulation to determine the 'safe period' (Fig. 45)
- assessing the cervical mucus which becomes profuse and watery *(Spinbarkeit)* at ovulation.

The failure rates for these methods may be as high as 25 pregnancies per 100 women years.

Coitus interruptus (removal of the penis from the vagina before ejaculation) is a widely used method of contraception; not particularly effective.

Barrier methods

Condoms When used with a spermicide, e.g. Nonoxynol-9, condoms are effective, resulting in only 2–3 failures per 100 women years. Condoms also act as a physical barrier to the transmission of many sexually transmitted infections; female condoms are also available (Fig. 46).

Caps The diaphragm (Fig. 47) is the most commonly used; other types include cervical and vault caps. When used with spermicide, a diaphragm is as effective as a condom and spermicide. It consists of a thin latex rubber dome attached to a circular metal spring. The size required is determined during an examination. It should cover the cervix, with the anterior edge of the diaphragm lying behind the symphysis pubis and the posterior edge in the posterior fornix. It should be inserted prior to intercourse and should not be removed for at least 6 h afterwards.

Others Disposable sponges impregnated with Nonoxynol-9 are currently available, but they are expensive to buy and not very effective.

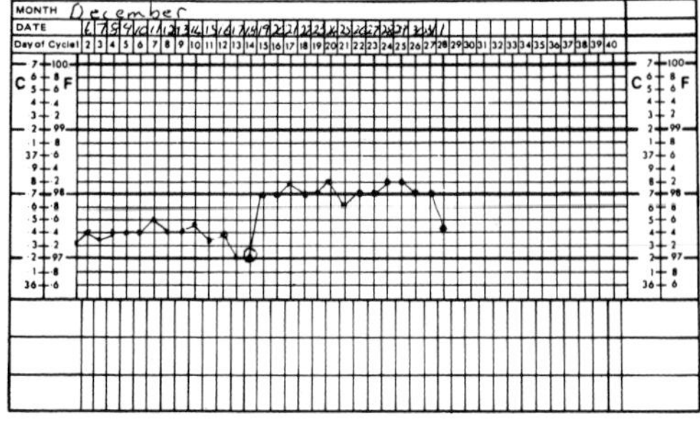

Fig. 45 Temperature chart – ovulatory biphasic pattern. Temperature rise follows ovulation and persists until just prior to menstruation.

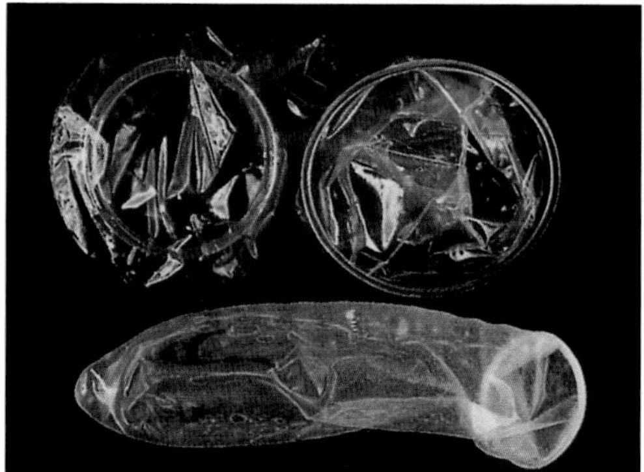

Fig. 46 Male and female condoms.

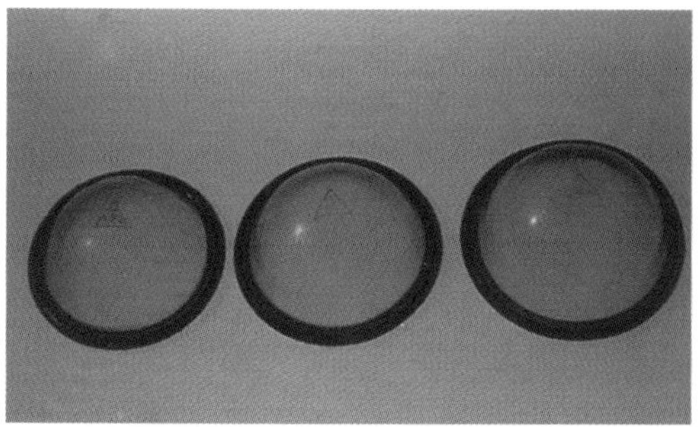

Fig. 47 Diaphragms.

Hormonal contraception

Combined oral contraceptive pills Contain both oestrogen and progesterone. They are taken cyclically for 21 days with a 7-day break. During the 'pill-free week', a withdrawal bleed is experienced. The combined pill acts on the hypothalamus and pituitary causing inhibition of GnRH, FSH and LH by negative feedback, thus preventing ovulation. The endometrium is also rendered unsuitable for implantation. The progesterone element of the combined pill makes the cervical mucus impenetrable to sperm and may also interfere with fallopian tube function. The combined pill should not be used by women with hormone-dependent tumours (breast, endometrium, trophoblast). Thromboembolism, arterial disease, valvular heart disease, focal migraine, clotting abnormalities and liver disease are all contraindications to pill usage. Smoking, hypertension and diabetes are considered 'relative contraindications'. The combined pill is the most effective reversible method of contraception currently available (Fig. 48).

Progesterone-only pills These do not necessarily inhibit ovulation; they act on the endometrium, the endocervical mucus and the fallopian tubes. Progesterone-only preparations should be taken at the same time every day, without any breaks. The maximal effect on cervical mucus is seen 4–6 h after taking the pills. Even with good compliance, progesterone-only pills are less effective than combined pills.

Depot progestogen injections Used in sufficiently high doses, these will:

- inhibit ovulation
- render the endometrium atrophic
- thicken the cervical mucus.

This form of contraception is effective, safe, convenient and reversible. Some women will, however, suffer from weight gain and bleeding irregularities.

Implants One rod of etonogestrel is inserted subdermally every 3 years (Fig. 49).

The Pearl index is used to rate the effectiveness of a contraceptive method and is defined as:

The number of women who will become pregnant if 100 women used that form of contraception properly according to instructions for one year (or the percentage of women experiencing an unwanted pregnancy in one year of use). This is distinct from the actual failure rate from 'typical use' rather than 'perfect use' of the method.

Method	Pearl index	Method	Pearl index
No contraception	80–90	Contraceptive patch	<1
Male condom	2	IUCD	1–2
Female condom	5	LNG-IUS	1
Diaphragm and cap	4–8	Natural family planning	2–6
COCP	<1	Persona	6
POP	1	Female sterilisation	0.5
Injectable progestagens	<1	Male sterilisation	0.05
Progestagen Implants	<1		

Fig. 48 The Pearl Index.

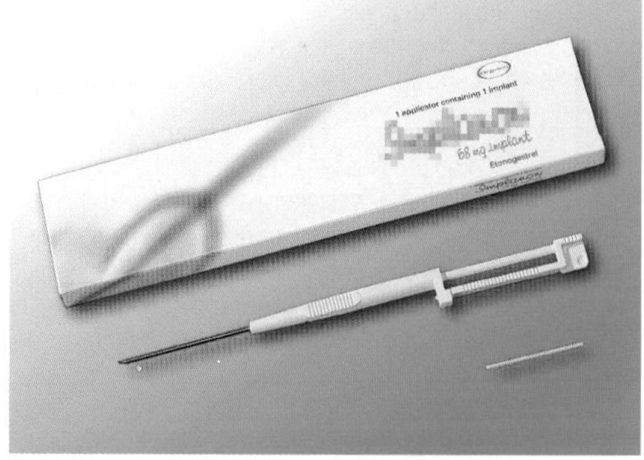

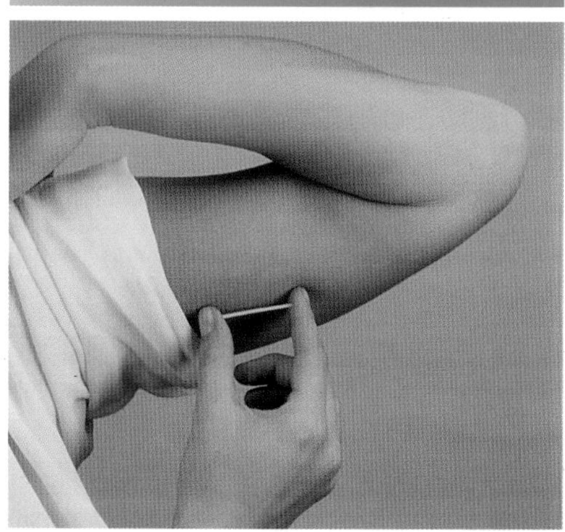

Fig. 49 Progesterone implant.

Postcoital contraception Two tablets each containing 750 mg of levonorgestrel. The first tablet must be taken within 72 h of unprotected intercourse and the second 12 h later. This regimen prevented 86% of expected pregnancies. Nausea may be experienced as a side effect.

Intrauterine contraceptive devices (IUCD)

The IUCD (Fig. 50) is placed in the uterus by a doctor using a sterile technique. It acts by altering/inhibiting sperm migration and ovum transport. The sterile inflammatory response to the presence of a foreign body inhibits implantation of the blastocyst. It is a safe, highly effective and reversible form of contraception, but it must be fitted by a doctor and requires follow-up care. An IUCD should not be fitted in women who have had pelvic inflammatory disease, or if there is an intrauterine pregnancy or uterine abnormality. It can be used as a method of postcoital contraception. To be effective if must be fitted within 5 days of unprotected intercourse.

Progesterone releasing intrauterine system (IUS)

Progestogens are released into the uterine cavity and prevent proliferation and cause thickening of the cervical mucus. The devices also reduce menstrual blood loss and dysmenorrhoea. They are one of the most effective reversible methods of contraception.

Sterilization

Female methods of sterilization involve the blockage of the fallopian tubes. This can be achieved by excision or occlusion with clips (Fig. 51), rings, or by diathermy via the laparoscope or a mini-laparotomy. It is highly effective and should be considered irreversible. The failure rate is about 0.1%.

Male sterilization is a good alternative to female sterilization and should be discussed with couples presenting to the gynaecology clinic requesting sterilization.

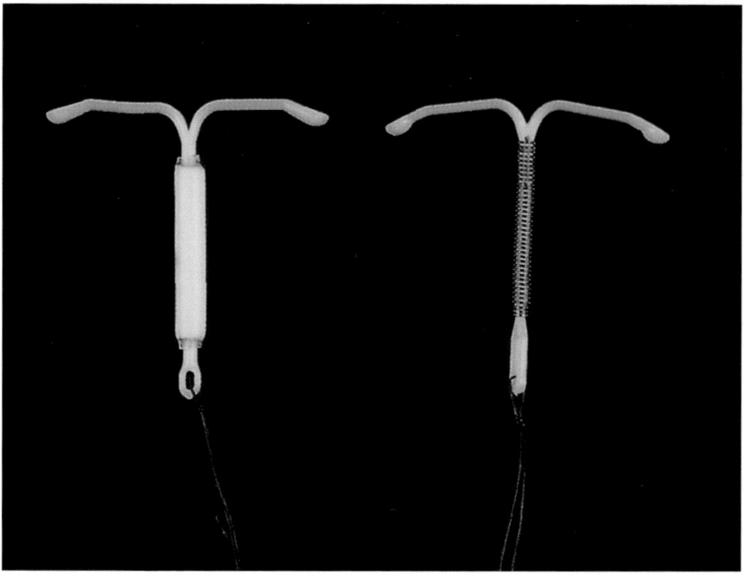

Fig. 50 Intrauterine contraceptive devices: (left) Progestagen-containing IUS; (right) Nova T IUCD.

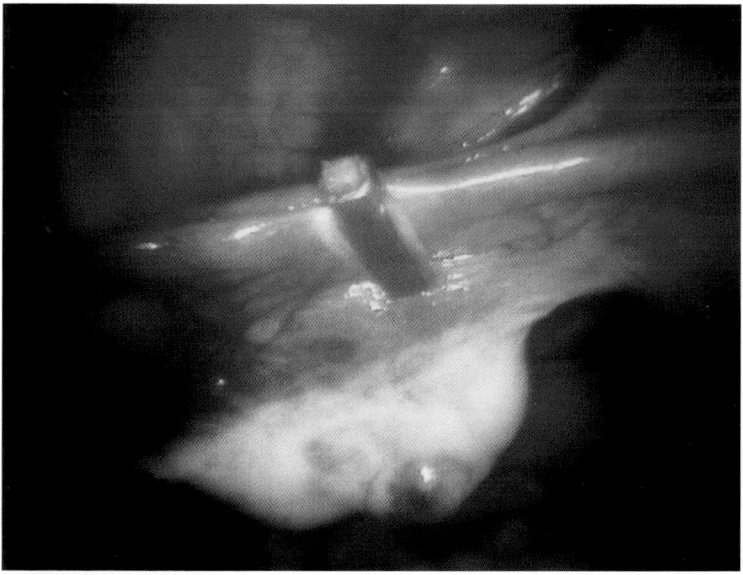

Fig. 51 Sterilization clip.

6 Early pregnancy problems

Miscarriage

Definition

A spontaneous loss of pregnancy before 24 weeks.

Incidence

15–25% of all pregnancies end in miscarriage.

Classification

Miscarriage can be classified as follows (Fig. 52):

- *Threatened miscarriage:* fetus is still viable, and the cervical os is closed.
- *Inevitable miscarriage:* fetus may still be alive but the cervical os is open.
- *Incomplete miscarriage:* some products of conception have been expelled already.
- *Complete miscarriage:* fetus and placental tissue have all been expelled.
- *Delayed miscarriage:* the pregnancy has succumbed but has not been expelled (Fig. 52).

Aetiology

The majority of miscarriages are due to chromosomal defects. If they are in the first trimester it is not necessarily helpful investigating women who miscarry – unless they have had three consecutive spontaneous miscarriages. The causes can be:

- abnormal conceptus (chromosomal or structural)
- immunological
- uterine abnormality
- cervical incompetence
- endocrine
- maternal disease (including systemic lupus erythematosus)
- infection
- toxins and cytotoxic drugs
- trauma.

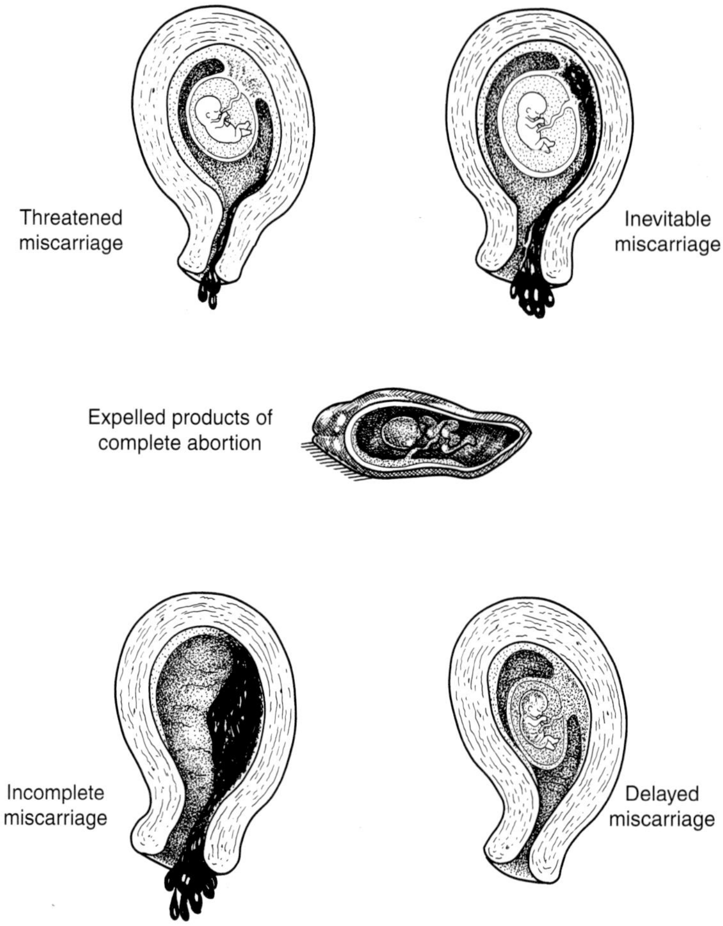

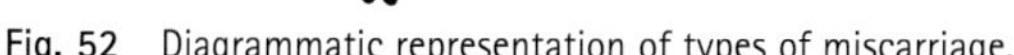

Fig. 52 Diagrammatic representation of types of miscarriage.

Clinical features

Patients will present with amenorrhoea followed by vaginal bleeding. Pain may be present. The symptoms of pregnancy may have disappeared. On examination there may be lower abdominal tenderness. The bleeding may vary from spotting to heavy bleeding. The uterine size may be smaller than dates (if products have been expelled), the same size, or larger than dates (if bleeding has occurred into the uterine cavity). The cervix may be closed or open depending on the stage of the miscarriage.

Differential diagnosis

- Ectopic pregnancy
- Hydatidiform mole
- Dysfunctional uterine bleeding

Investigations

If the cervical os is open, the pregnancy will not continue and no further investigations are needed. If the os is closed, an ultrasound scan will determine whether a viable fetus is present in the uterine cavity (Fig. 53).

Management

There is no proven treatment for a threatened abortion. Inevitable, incomplete, complete and missed abortions all require evacuation of the uterus (Fig. 54).

Recurrent miscarriage

There is increasing evidence that women who recurrently miscarry may have anticardiolipin and antiphospholipid antibodies (antiphospholipid antibody syndrome). Women who have three or more miscarriages should be referred to a specialist unit where this can be investigated. Women with antiphospholipid antibody syndrome also appear to be at risk of later pregnancy problems including pre-eclampsia and intrauterine growth restriction. The treatment may include heparin and the use of low-dose aspirin from as soon as a viable pregnancy is diagnosed.

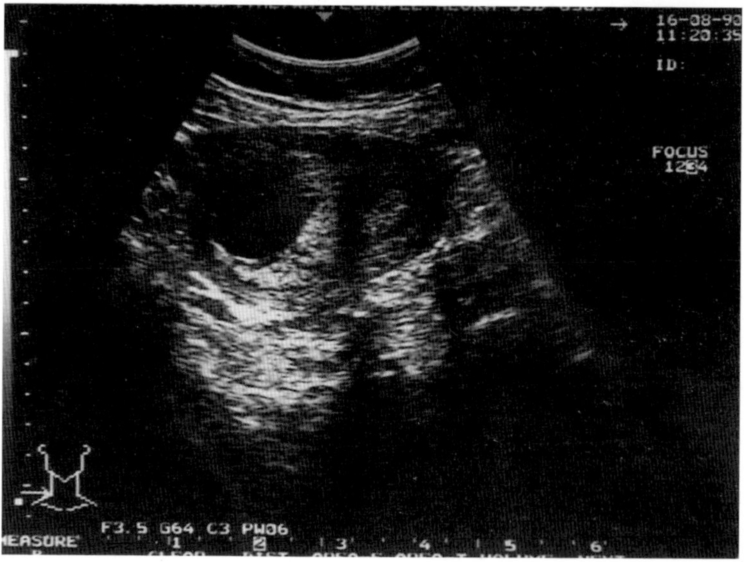

Fig. 53 Ultrasound picture of a delayed miscarriage in a bicornuate uterus.

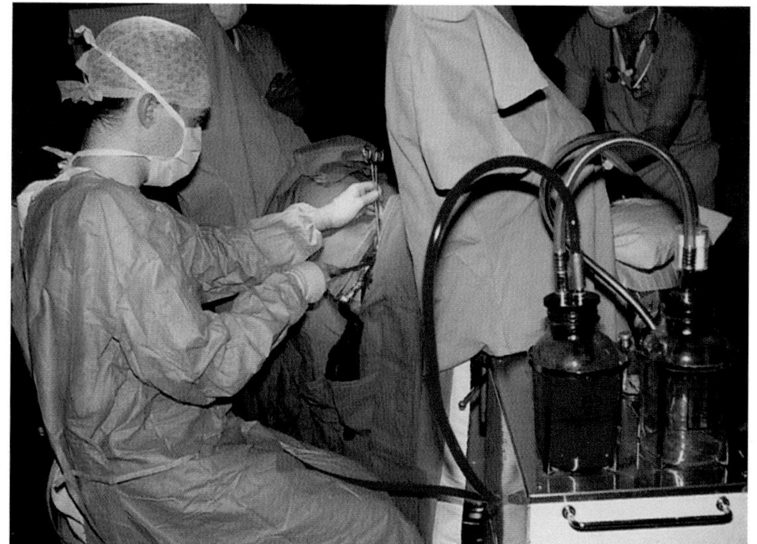

Fig. 54 Surgical evacuation of the uterus.

Ectopic pregnancy: diagnosis

Definition

The implantation of a pregnancy outside the uterine cavity (usually in the ampullary part of the fallopian tube).

Aetiology

Any factor that will decrease embryo transport along the tube can lead to an ectopic pregnancy. The most common cause is previous pelvic infection.

Patho-physiology

The fertilized ovum is delayed in its transport along the tube and implants on the tubal mucosa. Intratubal or intraperitoneal bleeding occurs as a result of erosion and distension of the tubal wall (Fig. 55). The uterine endometrium undergoes decidualization in response to the hormonal stimulus of the trophoblast.

Clinical features

Symptoms

Classically, the patient will have had amenorrhoea followed by irregular spotting or vaginal bleeding and unilateral pain (may be bilateral).

Signs

These will vary depending on whether tubal rupture has occurred. If tubal rupture has occurred the patient may be in shock.

The abdominal signs can vary from unilateral lower abdominal tenderness with rebound to a rigid abdomen with guarding. Vaginally there is usually cervical excitation, unilateral tenderness, and a mass may be felt on one side.

Differential diagnosis

- Miscarriage
- Pelvic infection

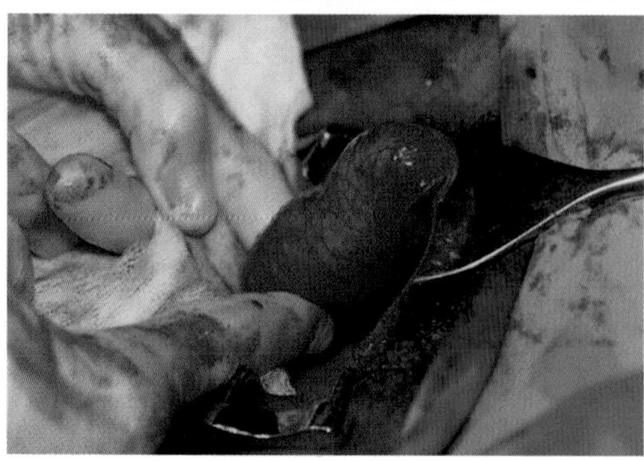

Fig. 55 Ectopic gestation distending the fallopian tube.

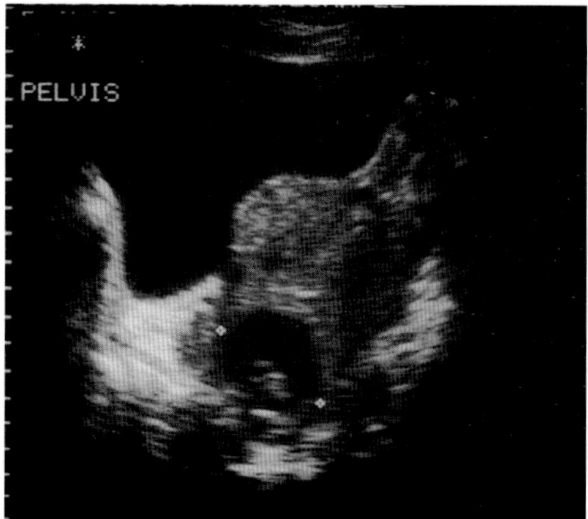

Fig. 56 Gestation sac lateral to the uterus that is indenting the bladder.

Ectopic pregnancy: Management

Investigations

Ultrasound scan is useful to confirm an intrauterine pregnancy, or an ectopic pregnancy can be seen outside the uterine cavity (see Fig. 56), and free fluid can be seen in the pouch of Douglas.

Blood sampling Quantitative HCG assay and FBC, and cross-matching.

Management

The quantitative HCG, the ultrasound findings and the clinical picture will determine whether conservative or interventional management is appropriate. If the level of HCG does not fall at an acceptable rate and/or the clinical situation is not resolving, then laparoscopy is mandatory.

Laparoscopy The fallopian tube may appear distended or filled with blood (Fig. 57) and/or there may be free blood in the pelvis. Laparoscopic salpingectomy (removal of the tube) is the treatment of choice if the other tube is laparoscopically normal.

Laparotomy Should be considered if the patient is in shock due to a ruptured ectopic pregnancy or any situation that can not be safely dealt with laparoscopically.

Occasionally a tubal abortion may have occurred and the fetus may be free in the peritoneal cavity (Fig. 58).

Prognosis

The intrauterine pregnancy rate after surgery is 50% and the repeat ectopic rate is 20%.

Only one-third of women will proceed to have a successful term baby.

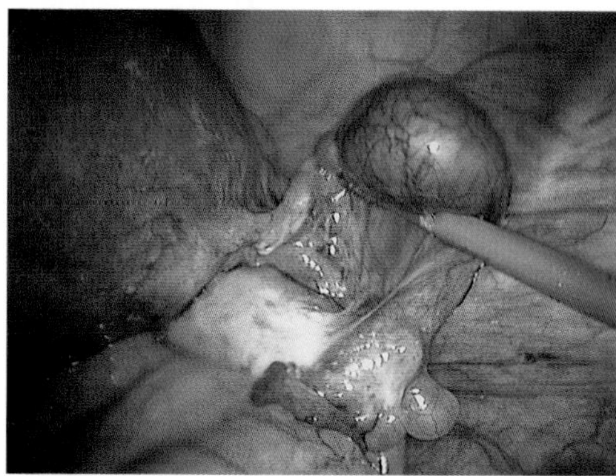

Fig. 57 Fallopian tube distended with blood as seen laparoscopically.

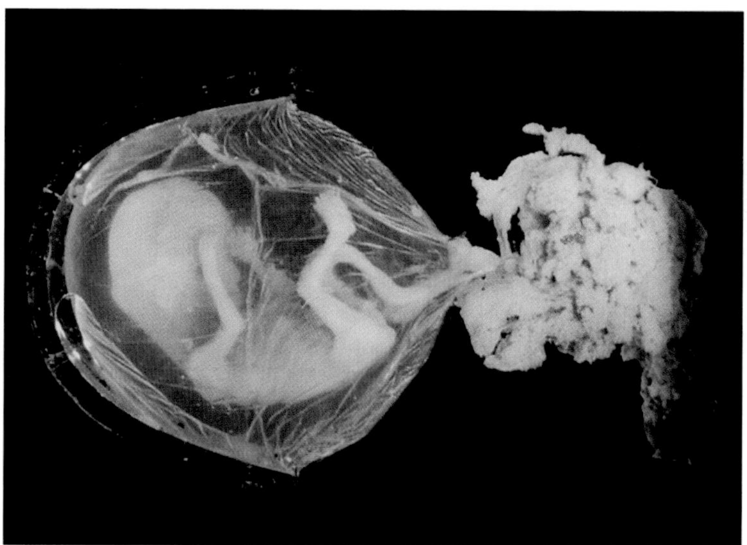

Fig. 58 Fetus found free in the peritoneal cavity.

Trophoblastic disease

Definition

Hydatidiform mole is a tumour of trophoblast.

Incidence

Varies geographically, with a higher incidence in Asiatic countries than in the West.

Aetiology

Unknown.

Classification

Complete mole No fetus is present and the chromosomal complement is totally paternal. There are 46 chromosomes.

Partial mole Fetus is present. There are 69 chromosomes and the extra set is of paternal origin.

Invasive mole May penetrate the uterus and/or metastasize to the lungs.

Clinical features

The symptoms are usually irregular bleeding in the first trimester of pregnancy. The uterus may be larger than dates and the fetal heart is usually absent. Pre-eclampsia may develop early, and theca lutein cysts may be palpable.

Investigations

Ultrasound will demonstrate a 'snowstorm' appearance, and the fetus will not be seen (Fig. 59). Beta-HCG level is very high. A chest X-ray should be done to exclude pulmonary metastases.

Management

Suction evacuation of the hydropic vesicles (Fig. 60). If uterine size is too large, extra-amniotic prostaglandins are used. Hysterectomy may be done in the older woman. It is essential to follow all women to ensure that the beta-HCG levels disappear.

Follow-up

This is co-ordinated through two centres in the UK. If the patient's HCG level reaches the normal range within 56 days of evacuation, follow-up is limited to 6 months, during which time the patients are advised not to conceive. If the HCG has not returned to normal within 8 weeks of evacuation, follow-up is for 2 years.

Prognosis

One in 30 moles develops into choriocarcinoma—a malignant tumour of trophoblastic tissue. Chemotherapy is the mainstay of treatment and close follow-up is essential.

In subsequent pregnancies women must attend early to exclude molar pregnancy by ultrasound and an HCG should be performed 3 weeks after delivery.

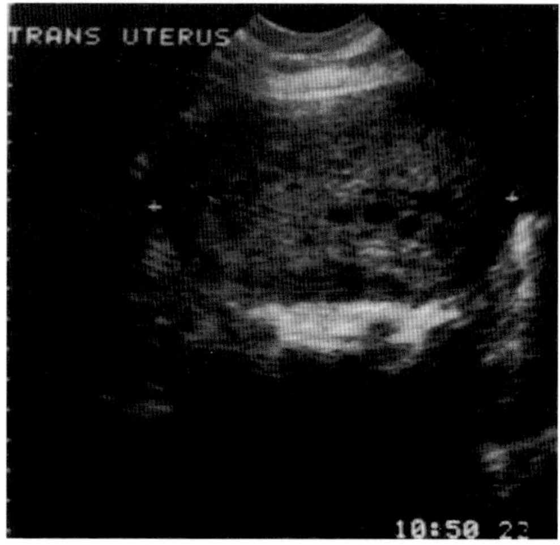

Fig. 59 Ultrasound picture of hydatidiform mole.

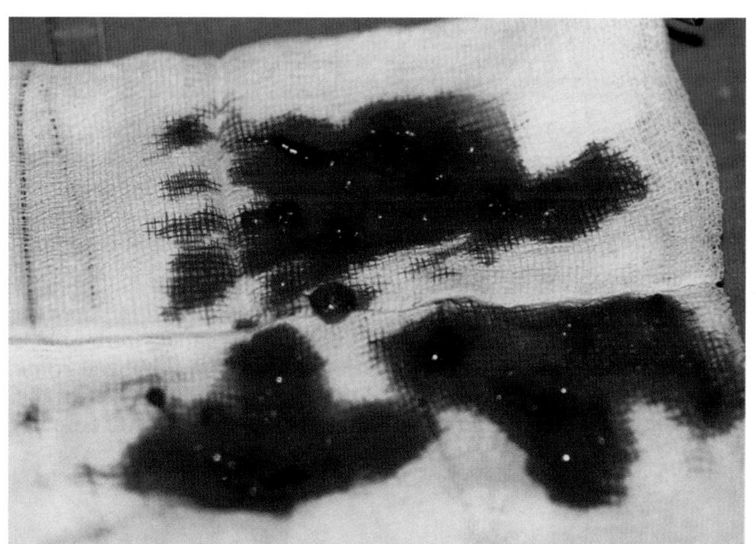

Fig. 60 Hydropic vesicles of hydatidiform mole.

7 Therapeutic abortion

Definition

Medical termination of pregnancy prior to 24 weeks' gestation.

Classification

Terminations can be performed for fetal or maternal reasons. Most are performed because the continuation of the pregnancy will cause risk to the physical or mental health of the woman.

Investigations

If gestation is in doubt, an ultrasound scan should be performed. Full blood count, blood group, Rhesus status and haemoglobin electrophoresis should be undertaken if indicated.

Management

Counselling is essential in pregnancy termination. The appropriate forms (Fig. 61) must be filled out with two certifying practitioners. The method of termination will depend on the gestation.

Progesterone antagonists These are used in combination with a prostaglandin pessary prior to 9 weeks' gestation, leading to a 'medical' termination of pregnancy.

Dilatation and evacuation The cervix is dilated (this can be made easier if a prostaglandin pessary is used prior to surgery) and then the uterine contents are removed, usually with a suction curettage (up to 14 weeks' gestation).

Prostaglandins Labour is induced with prostaglandins after 14 weeks' gestation. They can be administered as vaginal pessaries, intra-amniotically or extra-amniotically. Whatever the route, the procedure is followed by an evacuation of the uterus to ensure that the uterine cavity is empty. Mifepristone and gemeprost are becoming more popular.

IN CONFIDENCE **ABORTION NOTIFICATION**

Please leave blank

ABORTION ACT 1967
FORM OF NOTIFICATION (England and Wales)

This form is to be COMPLETED BY THE PRACTITIONER TERMINATING THE PREGNANCY and sent in a sealed envelope within SEVEN DAYS of the termination to:-

The Chief Medical Officer
Department of Health
Richmond House
79 Whitehall
LONDON
SW1A 2NS

OR

The Chief Medical Officer
Welsh Office
Cathays Park
CARDIFF
CF1 3NQ

in respect of the termination of the pregnancy in Wales

PLEASE USE BLOCK CAPITALS AND NUMERALS FOR DATES THROUGHOUT

1. PRACTITIONER TERMINATING THE PREGNANCY

NAME I, ...

PERMANENT ADDRESS of ....

....

hereby give notice that I terminated the pregnancy of the woman named overleaf, and to the best of my knowledge the particulars on this form are correct. **I further certify that I joined/did not join† in giving Certificate A having seen/not seen† and examined/not examined† her before doing so.**

Signature .... **Date** ....

2. CERTIFICATION In all non-emergency cases state particulars of practitioners who joined in giving Certificate A.

1. To be completed in **all** cases.

2. Do **not** complete if the operating practitioner joined in giving Certificate A.

NAME ....

PERMANENT ADDRESS ....

....

(tick appropriate box)

Did the practitioner named at 1 certify that he saw/and examined the pregnant woman before giving the certificate? ☐ YES ☐ NO

Did the practitioner named at 2 certify that he saw/and examined the pregnant woman before giving the certificate? ☐ YES ☐ NO

DO NOT COMPLETE IF SECTION 20 BELOW APPLIES

Please leave these boxes blank

3. NAME AND ADDRESS OF PLACE OF TERMINATION ....

....

(tick appropriate box)

Was the patient a NHS case terminated in an approved place under an agency agreement? ☐ YES ☐ NO ☐

† delete as appropriate

Form HSA4 (Revised 1991)

Fig. 61 'Yellow form'. (Crown copyright. Reproduced by permission.)

8 Gynaecological infections

Lower genital tract infections

The most common manifestations are vaginal discharge and vulvovaginitis.

Candida (thrush)

Aetiology

Most cases are due to *Candida albicans* (a yeast-like fungus). Yeasts may be present in the vagina without causing symptoms. Candida is not necessarily sexually transmitted, it can spread from the anus to the vulva and vagina. Once established, however, it can be transmitted sexually even by an asymptomatic partner.

Clinical features

Yeasts are the most common cause of vaginitis and vaginal discharge. The discharge is characteristically white, particulate, non-offensive and irritant. The vulva may appear red and oedematous and/or covered in white discharge (Fig. 62). In the vagina, white discharge (the texture of cottage cheese) adheres to the vaginal walls (Fig. 63). Yeasts can be identified by microscopy and Gram staining of a high vaginal swab, and by culture in the appropriate medium.

Management

Treatment includes topical antifungal agents, pessaries and creams. Severe cases may require systemic therapy with oral antifungal agents, e.g. fluconazole.

Trichomonas vaginalis (TV)

Aetiology

TV is a flagellate parasite found in the vagina, the urethra (of both men and women) and in the upper genital tract. It is the second most common cause of vaginal discharge. It is sexually acquired and is often found in association with gonorrhoea. The vaginal discharge is thin, yellow, offensive and irritant, often appearing frothy and causing reddening of the vaginal epithelium and the cervix (see Fig. 64). The organism is identified by microscopy of a high vaginal sample mixed with a drop of saline.

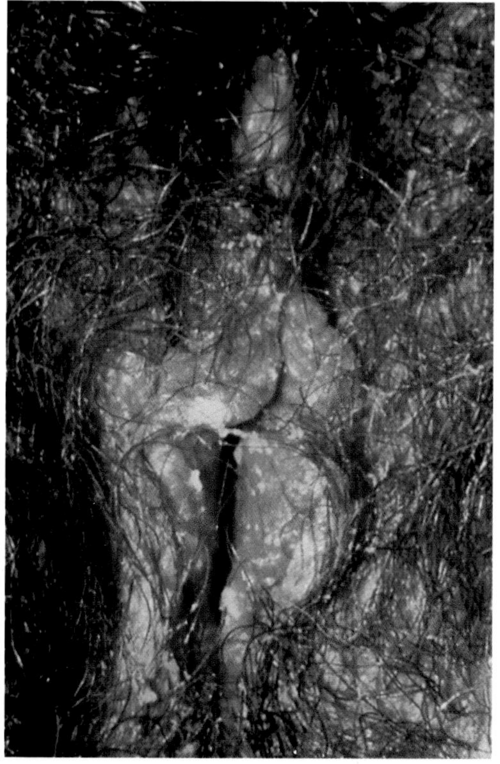

Fig. 62 Vulval candidiasis.

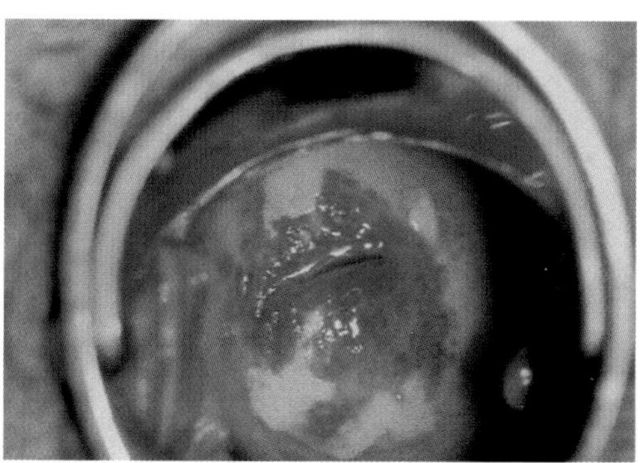

Fig. 63 Vaginal candidiasis.

Bacterial vaginosis
This is characterized by an offensive vaginal discharge that gives a positive amine test, has a pH greater than 5, and 'clue cells' seen on microscopy of a Gram stained smear. The cause is a mixed infection with *Gardnerella vaginalis* and anaerobic organisms including *Bacteroides* species and *Peptostreptococcus.*
Treatment is with oral metronidazole or clindamycin cream.
Other causes of vaginal discharge include increased but normal vaginal secretion, e.g. at ovulation, during sexual excitement or during pregnancy, and abnormal discharge due to chemical irritants, foreign bodies or degenerative conditions.

Warts (human papilloma virus: HPV)

Description

Warts are caused by the human papilloma virus. They can be flat and undetectable to the naked eye, or large exophytic lesions. The cervix (Fig. 65), vaginal and vulval surfaces (Fig. 66) are all susceptible to infection. HPV has been strongly implicated as a causative factor in cervical neoplasia. The incubation period varies from 3 weeks to 8 months. It may present as painless slow-growing vulvovaginal lumps. The differential diagnoses include molluscum contagiosum (caused by a pox virus) condylomata lata (lesions of secondary syphylis) and other skin tags, naevi or sebaceous cysts.

Management

The following treatments are available: podophyllin (a cytotoxic agent), trichloracetic acid, electrocautery, cryocautery and excision. The last three are reserved for resistant and extensive warts. Barrier contraception is advised.

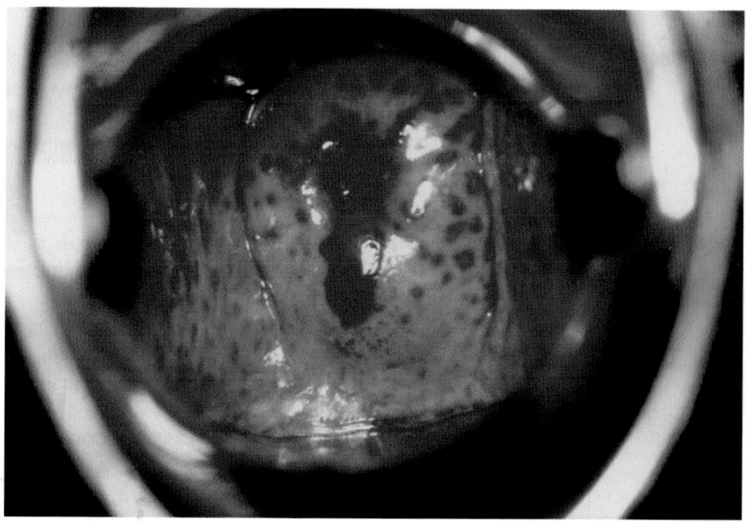

Fig. 64 Trichomonal 'strawberry cervix'.

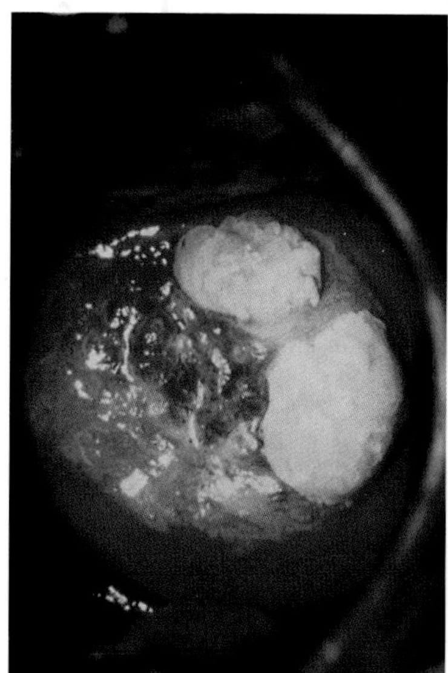

Fig. 65 Cervical warts.

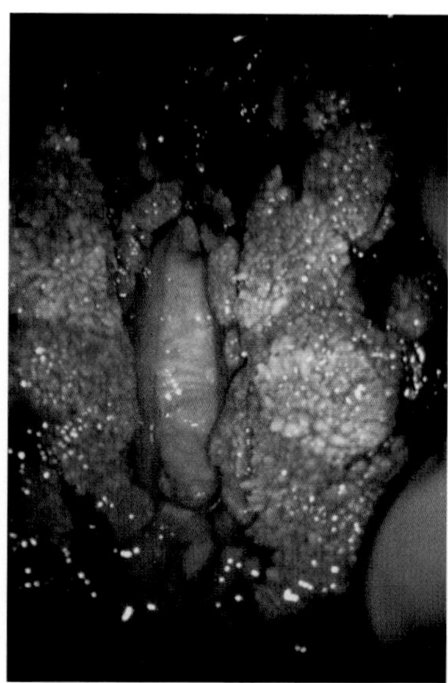

Fig. 66 Florid vulval warts.

Herpes simplex virus (HSV)

Aetiology

Genital and anal herpes is usually caused by type II HSV, but type I HSV (usually responsible for oral cold sores) can also be a cause of genital infection. In the UK, genital HSV is the most common identifiable cause of genital ulceration.

Clinical features

A primary infection may present with prodromal discomfort, followed by the appearance of vesicles (Fig. 67), ulceration, inguinal lymphadenopathy together with malaise, fever and possibly urinary retention. In women the vesicles are usually situated on the vulva (Fig. 68), vagina and cervix. The lesions of a primary infection may take several weeks to heal and secondary infection is common. Recurrence of HSV infection is common, as the virus lies dormant in the posterior nerve root ganglia between recurrences. Recurrent infection is less florid. Diagnosis is made on clinical examination and confirmed by viral cultures from the ulcers.

Management

Aciclovir can be used to reduce symptoms and virus shedding times in a primary attack. It does not prevent recurrences except during continuous treatment.

Complications

Primary infection can give rise to systemic complications, including hepatitis, myelitis, encephalitis and meningitis. A primary infection in early pregnancy may cause abortion. Infection near term may be transmitted to the baby during delivery, leading to a high mortality rate and a high rate of neurological complications in the survivors. Primary infection or active recurrent disease at term are indications for delivery by caesarean section before rupture of the membranes.

Other pathogens

Chlamydia trachomatis and *Neisseria gonorrhoeae* infect the cervix and urethra. They are usually asymptomatic in the absence of spread to the upper genital tract.

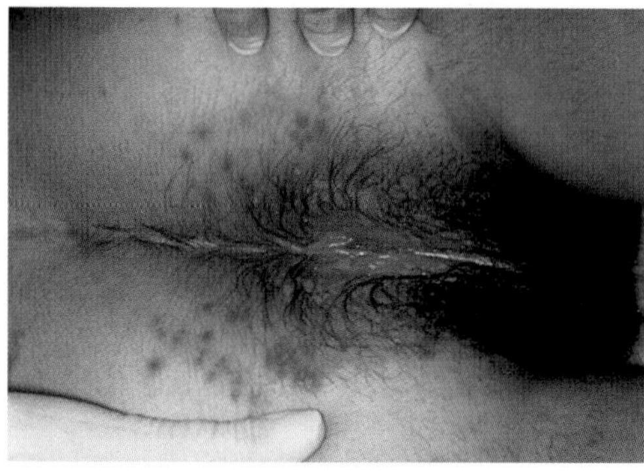

Fig. 67 Primary genital herpes infection.

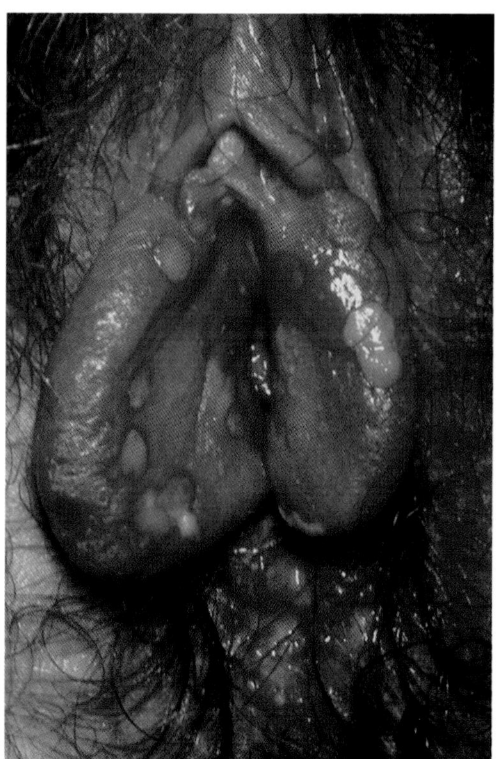

Fig. 68 Vulval herpes infection.

Pelvic inflammatory disease

Definition

An infection of the endometrium, fallopian tubes and/or contiguous structures caused by the ascent of microorganisms from the lower genital tract.

Incidence

Roughly 100 000 women in the UK develop PID each year. Most are less than 25 years of age.

Aetiology

The majority of cases of PID in young women are associated with sexually transmitted bacteria, e.g. *Chlamydia trachomatis* and *Neisseria gonorrhoeae*. These bacteria may initiate the process and then be replaced by opportunistic bacteria including streptococci and *Bacteroides*.

Clinical features

There is a spectrum of presentation from silent infection to florid symptoms and signs, e.g. pelvic pain, dyspareunia, fever, vaginal discharge, pyrexia, pelvic peritonism, cervical excitation and, possibly, a pelvic mass. Right upper quadrant pain may be due to perihepatitis (Fig. 69). It complicates up to 15% of cases of chlamydial PID. Laparoscopic evidence of PID (Fig. 70) is seen in only 65% of suspected cases.

Differential diagnosis

This includes acute appendicitis, endometriosis, ectopic pregnancy, ovarian cyst accident and inflammatory bowel conditions.

Management

A combination of antibiotics active against all likely causative organisms, along with adequate analgesia, are required. In severe cases, hospital admission may be necessary. Surgery is appropriate if the condition fails to improve or deteriorates with conservative management. All women with PID and their partners should be referred to a genitourinary medicine clinic, screened for sexually transmitted infections and treated appropriately to avoid reinfection.

Complications

Infertility follows in 15–20% of cases. There is a seven- to 10-fold increased risk of an ectopic pregnancy, and chronic pelvic pain is suffered by roughly 20% of women after PID.

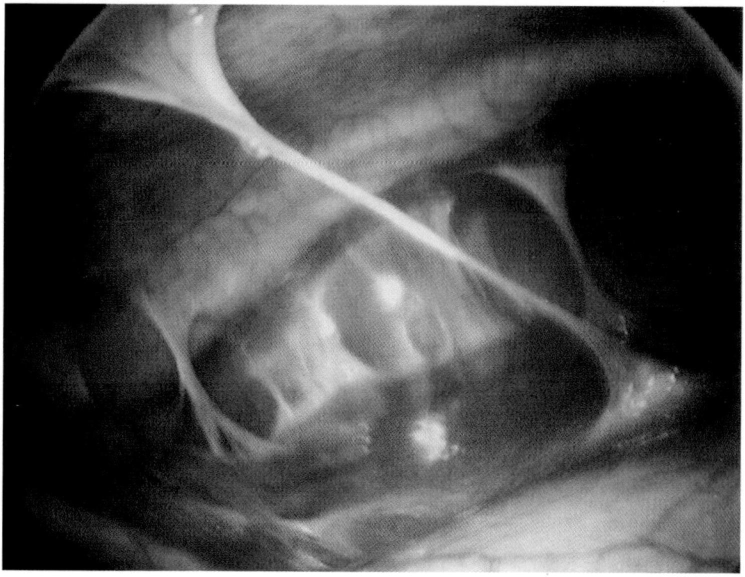

Fig. 69 Perihepatic adhesions (Fitz-Hugh-Curtis syndrome).

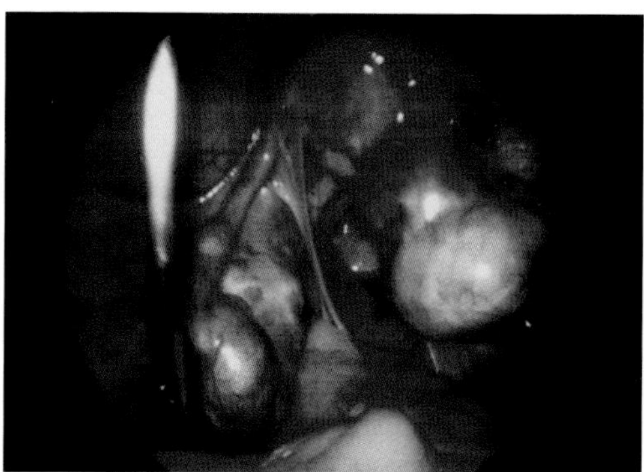

Fig. 70 Bilateral tubo-ovarian abscesses in PID.

HIV infection

Incidence and aetiology

HIV (human immunodeficiency virus) is most prevalent in North and South America, sub-Saharan Africa and western Europe. The age and sex distribution varies widely.

Mode of transmission

Sexual Heterosexual intercourse is the most common mode of transmission/acquisition world wide. In Europe and North America, women are accounting for an increasing proportion of new cases.

Parenteral Spread is from blood and blood products, before screening and heat treatment were introduced in 1985, and from sharing infected needles.

Transmission from mother to fetus 11–30% of children born to HIV-antibody-positive women will be infected (i.e. have antibodies persisting for more than 18 months or develop clinical and or immunological manifestations of HIV at an earlier stage). Maternal health is an important factor in transmission of infection to the fetus. Of those infants who acquire HIV from their mothers, about 25% will develop AIDS in the first year of life.

Clinical features

AIDS is defined as an illness caused by HIV and characterized by one or more 'indicator' diseases, which include candidiasis of the gastrointestinal (Fig. 71) and respiratory tract, cryptosporidiosis, *Pneumocystis carinii* pneumonia (Fig. 72) and toxoplasmosis of the brain (Fig. 73). Kaposi's sarcoma (Fig. 74) is rare in women; otherwise the spectrum of disease seen in men and women is similar.

Women and HIV

Important issues for women with HIV concern choice of contraception and wishes regarding pregnancy. There is no evidence that pregnancy accelerates the progress to AIDS. It has been suggested that the combined oral contraceptive pill may increase the risk of transmission and that an IUCD may put women with HIV at increased risk of pelvic inflammatory disease.

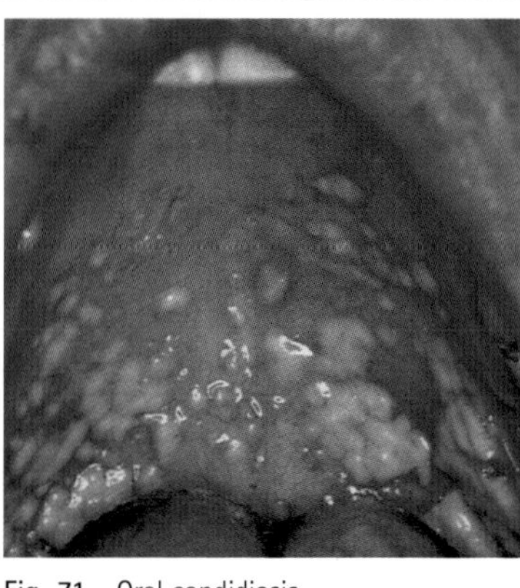

Fig. 71 Oral candidiasis.

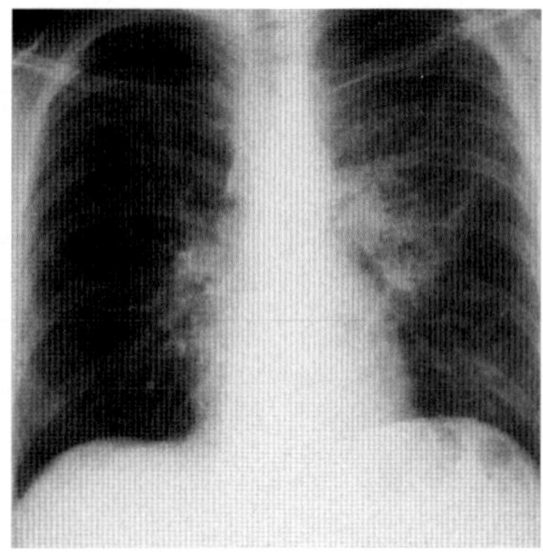

Fig. 72 *Pneumocystis carinii* pneumonia.

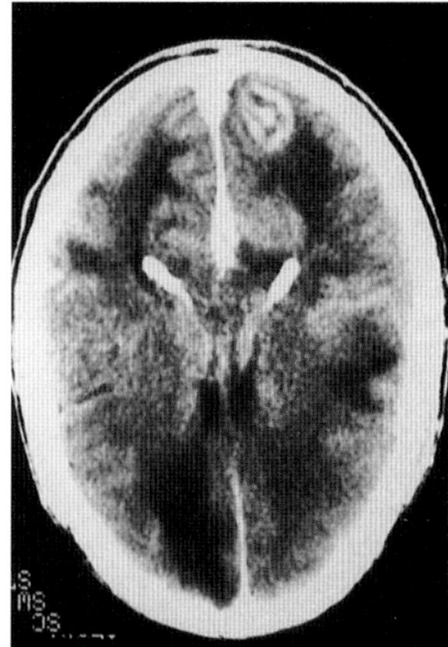

Fig. 73 Cerebral toxoplasmosis.

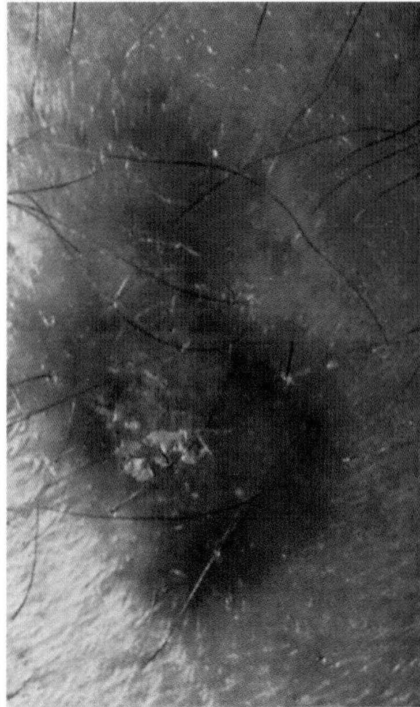

Fig. 74 Kaposi's sarcoma.

9 Endometriosis

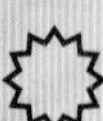

Definition

Endometriosis is a benign process characterized by the presence and proliferation of endometrial tissue in sites outside the uterine cavity.

Incidence

It is seen in up to 10% of premenopausal Caucasian women and 30% of women presenting with infertility. The use of the oral contraceptive pill reduces the incidence of endometriosis.

Aetiology

A number of theories regarding the pathogenesis of endometriosis exist, but no single theory will explain all cases. The condition may therefore result from a combination of the following:

- *Retrograde menstruation:* the passage of endometrial tissue along the fallopian tubes during menstruation with implantation in the peritoneal cavity
- *Lymphatic or vascular spread:* endometrial tissue embolizing to distant sites
- *Metaplasia of coelomic epithelium:* the repeated inflammatory insult from menstrual blood in the peritoneal cavity may lead to redifferentiation of the peritoneal tissue and the development of viable endometrial tissue

Pathology

A non-infectious process of inflammation, fibrosis and adhesion formation. The gross appearance is of black spots ('powder burns') (Fig. 75), commonly on the ovaries, uterosacral ligaments (Fig. 76) and pouch of Douglas. Adhesion formation and distortion of normal anatomy may be a feature in severe disease (Fig. 77). If the ovaries are involved, 'chocolate cysts' may form. Unusual sites for endometriosis include the umbilicus, laparotomy scars, episiotomy scars, cervix, bowel, bladder, lung, thigh and vulva.

Clinical features

These include pain, which may be cyclical, dyspareunia, backache and secondary dysmenorrhoea. Rarely there may be haematuria or rectal bleeding if the bladder or bowel are involved. Endometriosis may also be symptomless.

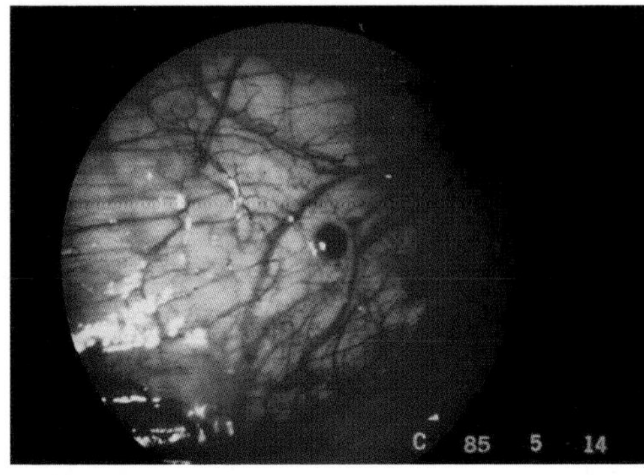

Fig. 75 Endometriotic deposit.

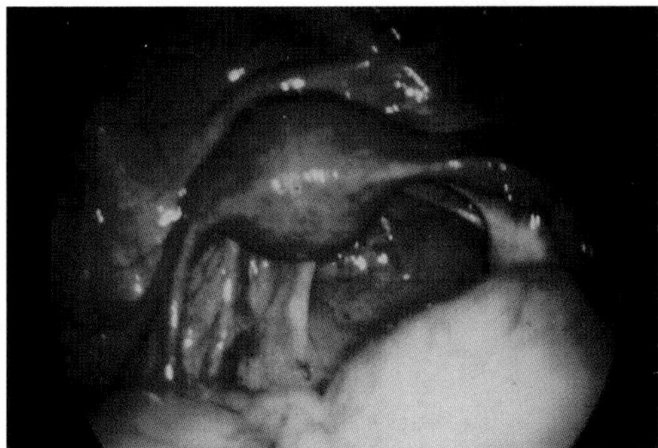

Fig. 76 Laparoscopy showing minimal endometriosis on left.

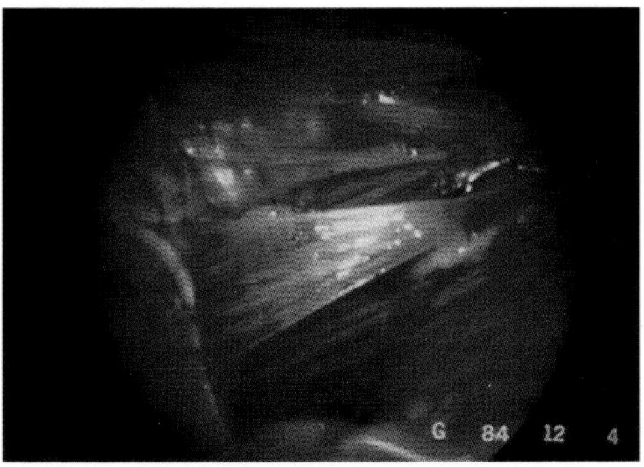

Fig. 77 Adhesions secondary to endometriosis.

Examination

A thorough clinical examination is essential and may reveal localized endometrial deposits, e.g. cervical endometriosis (Fig. 78).

Investigations

The definitive diagnosis is made by laparoscopy (Fig. 79) or laparotomy. If haematuria or rectal bleeding are features, cystoscopy, sigmoidoscopy and barium enema would be necessary.

Management

Symptomatic disease can be treated medically or surgically.

Medical treatment

Medicial treatment is based on the observation that endometriosis improves in pregnancy. The use of the oral contraceptive pill, without breaks for withdrawal bleeds, for up to 9 months mimics pregnancy and is associated with symptomatic improvement. Progestogens, e.g. medroxyprogesterone acetate, also suppress ovulation and give relief from symptoms. Danazol (a testosterone derivative) creates a high-androgen, low-oestrogen environment that does not support the growth of endometrium. Gestrinone acts similarly to danazol and has the advantage of being taken twice weekly as opposed to twice daily. GnRH analogues given intranasally or subcutaneously suppress ovulation at the hypothalamus.

Many medical treatments are effective in the treatment of endometriosis but unfortunately the condition can relapse. Side effects arise with all medications: breakthrough bleeding on the oral contraceptive pill; bloating and PMS-like symptoms with progestogen; androgenic side effects with danazol; and hypooestrogenic effects such as hot flushes and bone loss with GnRH analogues. (These can be counteracted with 'add-back' therapy.) Medical treatment must be tailored to the individual patient.

Surgical treatment

Surgical approaches can be through the laparoscope (diathermy or laser ablation and division of adhesions) or by laparotomy to restore pelvic anatomy or remove the uterus and ovaries.

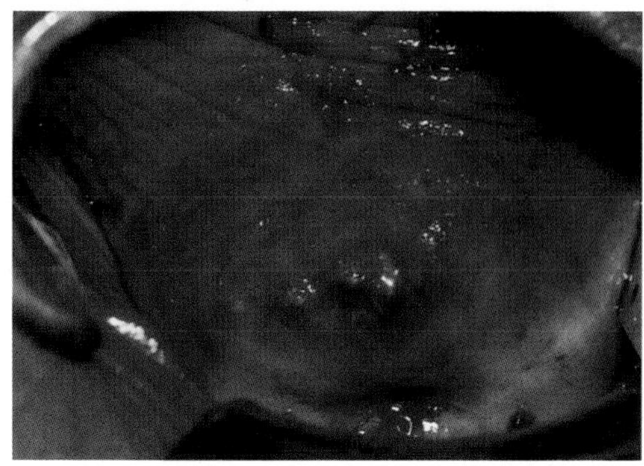

Fig. 78 Cervical endometriosis.

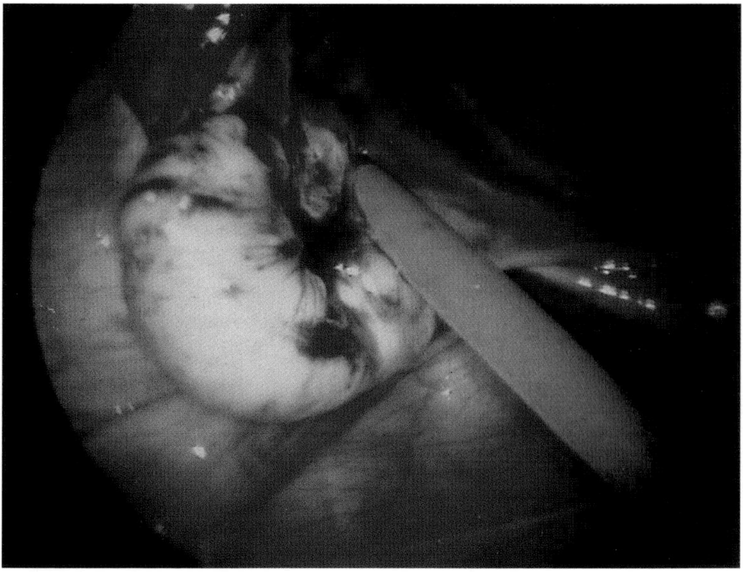

Fig. 79 Laparoscopic division of endometriotic adhesion.

10 Infertility

Definition

Failure to conceive after 12 months of regular unprotected intercourse. 1:6 couples affected.

Aetiology

Three main causes of infertility: poor semen quality, tubal disorders and ovulatory disorders. Other rarer causes include mucus 'hostility' and sperm antibodies, impotence and retrograde ejaculation. This leaves a significant (10–20%) proportion with unexplained infertility, which includes psychological factors.

Clinical features

Significant clues to the aetiology can be achieved by a thorough history from both partners. In the female, evidence of ovulation can be gained from regularity of menstrual cycle and associated symptoms, e.g. mittleschmerz pain, cervical mucus changes and primary dysmenorrhoea.

Tubal disorders are usually the result of scarring and adhesions secondary to infection (Figs 80, 81) or pelvic surgery, e.g. ovarian cystectomy. In addition, endometriosis may cause pelvic scarring. If the distal portion of the tube is blocked, a hydrosalpinx may develop (Fig. 82). Tubal damage should be suspected if there is a history of IUCD use, PID, pelvic surgery or pelvic pain.

Examination may also reveal endocrinological disorders, e.g. PCOS, or the tissue atrophy of premature menopause, and physical signs of pelvic pathology, e.g. endometriotic scarring, ovarian cysts or fibroids.

In the male, history may reveal previous operations or infections. Stress and recent intercurrent illnesses may be associated with transitory reduced semen quality.

Examination should include testicles, looking for varicosities or the absence of the vas deferens. Reduced testicular size and increased firmness due to fibrosis may indicate spermatogenic failure. A swollen epididymis may indicate a blockage of the vas.

Rarely, azoospermia may be due to hypogonadotrophic hypogonadism, indicated by lack of secondary sexual development.

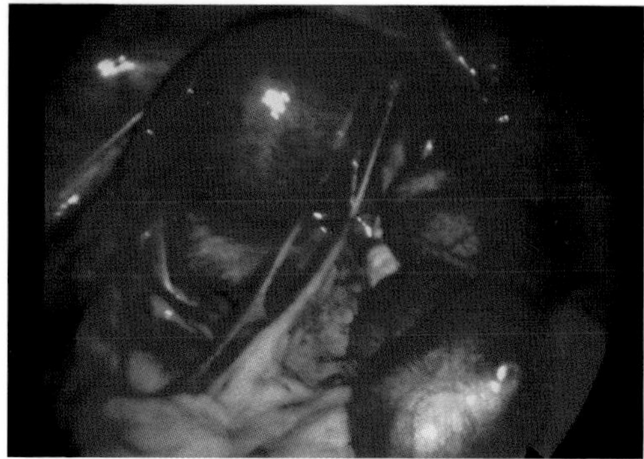

Fig. 80 Pelvic adhesions after PID.

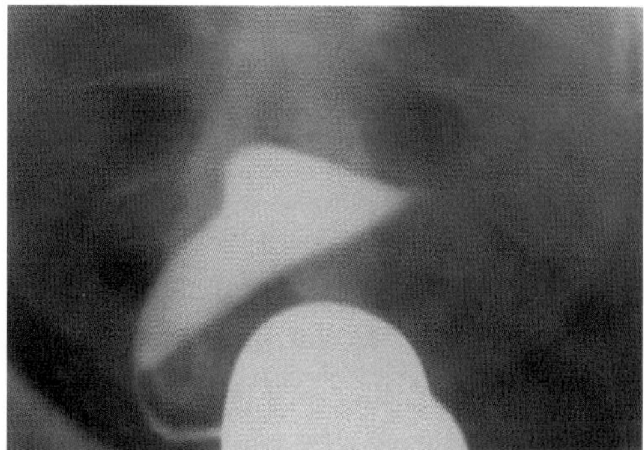

Fig. 81 Cornual blockage.

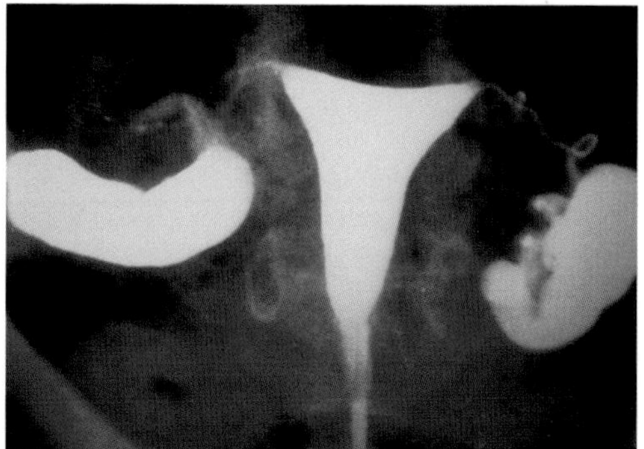

Fig. 82 Bilateral hydrosalpinges.

Differential diagnosis

Defining the specific causes of infertility requires a proper history and examination and appropriate investigations as outlined below.

Investigations

Male

For the male, a semen analysis on two occasions is the basic investigation. The WHO criteria for a normal semen analysis is a sperm density of ≥20 million sperm per mL with ≥50% sperm with forward progression and ≥50% normal morphology. The criteria are associated with a normal rate of conception. If the values are reduced, serum LH, FSH and testosterone are indicated. High gonadotrophins are indicative of testicular failure. Normal levels with reduced testosterone may indicate hypogonadotrophic hypogonadism. In cases of non-obstructive and some cases of obstructive azoospermia there may be an indication for testicular biopsy to assess spermatogenesis and storage of any sperm found for future use.

Female

In the female, simple tests for ovulation should be undertaken, i.e. mid-luteal phase serum progesterone, basal body temperature charts (Fig. 83) for no more than two cycles. More sophisticated investigations include follicle monitoring with ultrasound (Fig. 84), serial LH measurements to detect the pre-ovulatory LH surge, and laparoscopy in the luteal phase to confirm the presence of a corpus luteum.

Laparoscopy and dye instillation (Fig. 85) provide the optimum test of tubal patency or damage with the additional benefit of visualization of the pelvis, i.e. ovaries (for the presence of corpus luteum), peritoneum to exclude endometriotic deposits, and the uterus to assess anatomical abnormality. Hysterosalpingography is used to assess tubal patency and also to reveal intrauterine problems, e.g. adhesions, fibroids or anatomical abnormalities such as bicornuate uterus (Fig. 86). Other investigations include a postcoital test, which assesses the capacity of sperm to remain motile in the cervical mucus, and tests for antisperm antibodies in both partners and in the husband's seminal plasma.

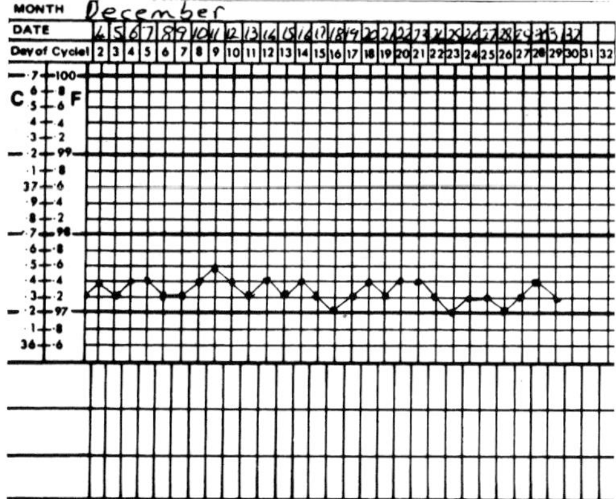

Fig. 83 Temperature chart showing an anovulatory pattern with absence of luteal phase rise.

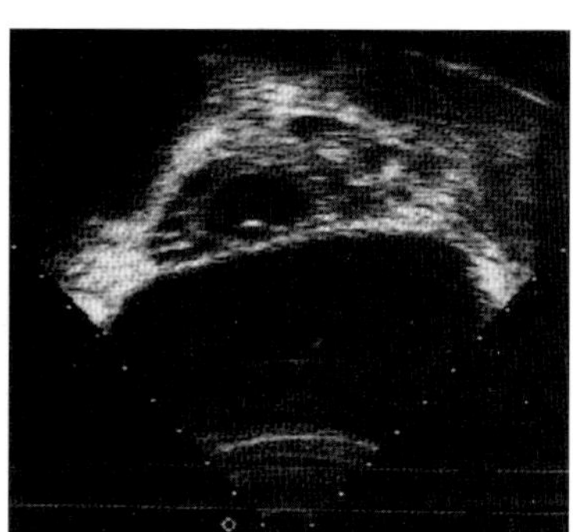

Fig. 84 Ultrasound image of a dominant follicle.

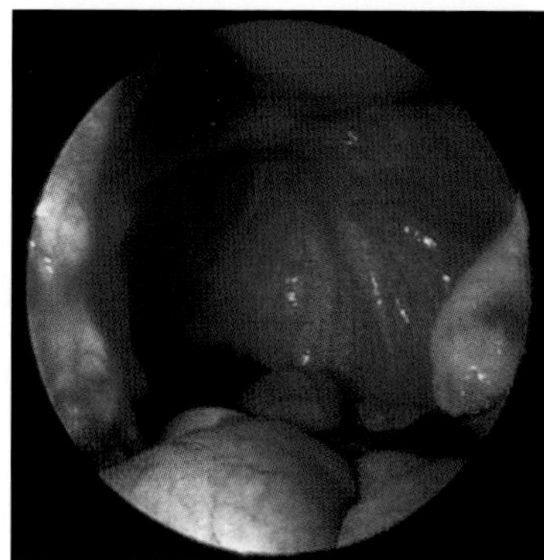

Fig. 85 Tubal patency as shown by presence of blue dye in the pelvis.

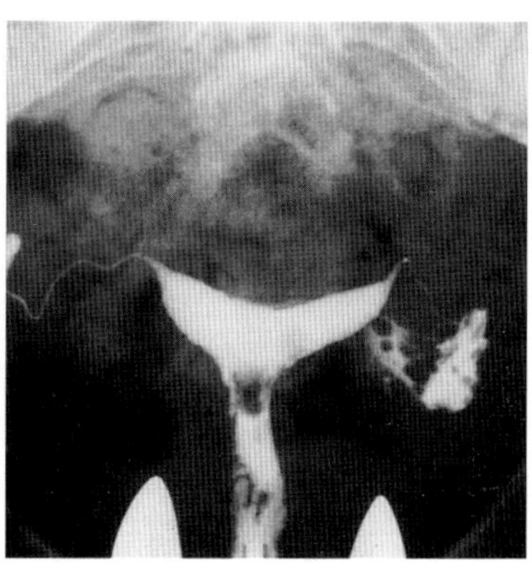

Fig. 86 Hysterosalpingogram of bicornuate uterus.

Management

Male

Poor semen quality previously had little opportunity for improvement unless it was a transitory problem, e.g. stress or viral infection. The value of varicocele repair is unresolved. Hormonal treatments are unproven. With low counts, options that are now available include the preparation of a small volume of the best sperm to place within the uterus at ovulation (intrauterine insemination; IUI) or in vitro fertilization (IVF) with oocytes collected from the patient. Intracytoplasmic sperm injection or ICSI has dramatically altered the treatment of severe male factor infertility. ICSI only requires low sperm numbers and can be used in the treatment of both obstructive and non-obstructive azoospermia. Antisperm antibodies have been successfully treated with steroids in the male. Donor semen remains the only option for many infertile men.

Female

Ovulatory disorders respond well to hormonal therapy, i.e. clomiphene or human menopausal gonadotrophins. The latter requires close monitoring to avoid hyperstimulation or high-order multiple pregnancy. Tubal damage can be dealt with by surgery (Fig. 87) in selected cases, but the results rarely exceed 30%.

Bypassing the tube with IVF is successful in 20–25% of cycles. This involves ovarian stimulation to produce multiple follicles, the aspiration of the oocytes from these follicles, the in vitro fertilization with partner's semen and transfer to the uterus 48–72 h after fertilization.

Assisted conception techniques including IVF and gamete intrafallopian transfer (GIFT: Fig. 88) are also applicable where mucus hostility is a possible cause or where no cause is found, e.g. unexplained infertility. Success rates in these groups are 25–30%.

Complications

The major complication of infertility other than those associated with drugs and surgical intervention is the psychological trauma of being unable to conceive. Significant morbidity is present in many couples, who require counselling and support to enable them to come to terms with childlessness.

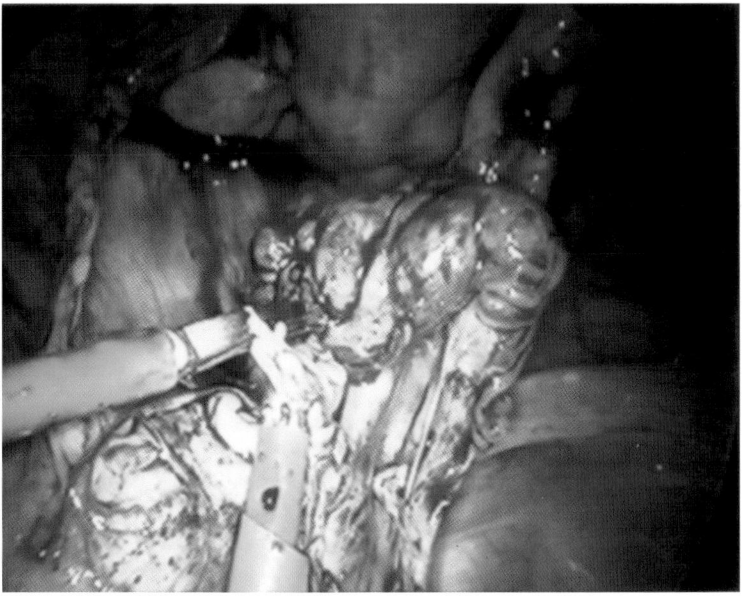

Fig. 87 Laparoscopic freeing of pelvic adhesions.

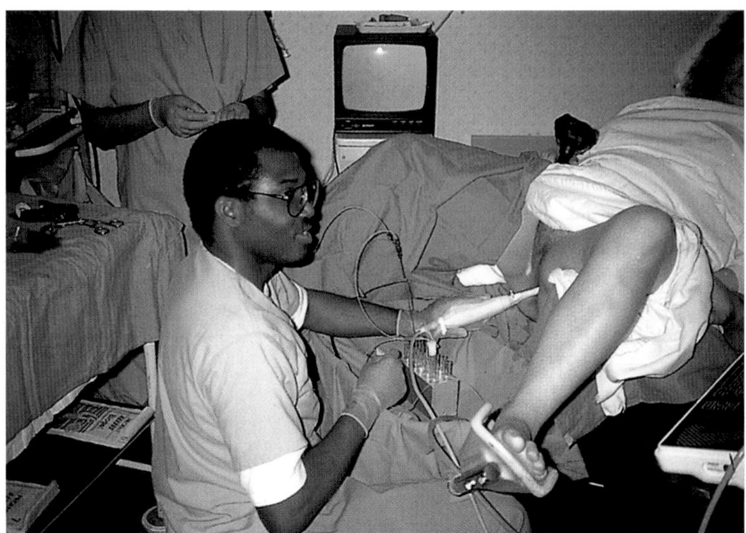

Fig. 88 Oocytes being aspirated for IVF.

11 Polycystic ovarian syndrome

Definition

Polycystic ovarian syndrome (PCOS) is a syndrome that consists of oligomenorrhoea, hirsutism (Figs 89, 90), obesity and infertility; it is associated with disordered pituitary gonadotrophin secretion and ovarian steroid production. It is a spectrum of disease as normally cycling women may have polycystic ovaries and yet none of the features above.

Incidence

Depending on the criteria used (clinical or ultrasound), the incidence varies from 5–30% of the female population. Amongst amenorrhoeic women, 30–40% probably have PCOS. Amongst hirsute women that incidence rises to 50–70%.

Aetiology

The cause of PCOS is uncertain. There are two main hypotheses:

- ovarian enzyme abnormality resulting in abnormal steroid production
- disordered feedback mechanisms acting on the pituitary, resulting in abnormal gonadotrophin secretion with secondary ovarian dysfunction

A small proportion of PCOS cases have been shown to be familial and due to ovarian enzyme abnormalities. The net result is an increased LH secretion, anovulation and increased ovarian androgen production.

Pathology

The classic polycystic ovary is increased in size due to:

- increased stromal tissue
- multiple ovarian cysts, 2–4 mm in diameter, distributed around the periphery of the ovary (pearl nodi; Fig. 91)

Clinical features

Obesity is usually present from childhood, while hirsutism usually appears at puberty, affecting the face, chest and abdomen. Oligomenorrhoea is present from puberty, often with episodes of secondary amenorrhoea. Infertility is usually primary.

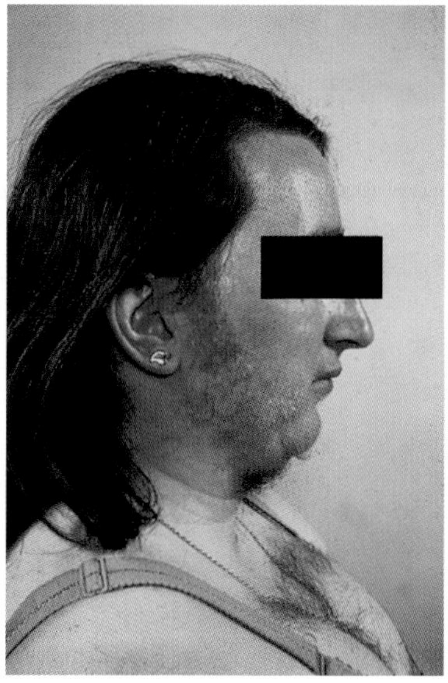

Fig. 89 Hirsutism before treatment.

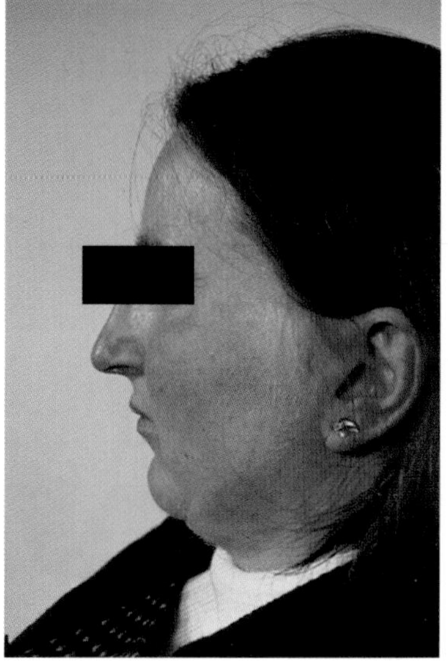

Fig. 90 Same patient as in Figure 89 after hormone treatment.

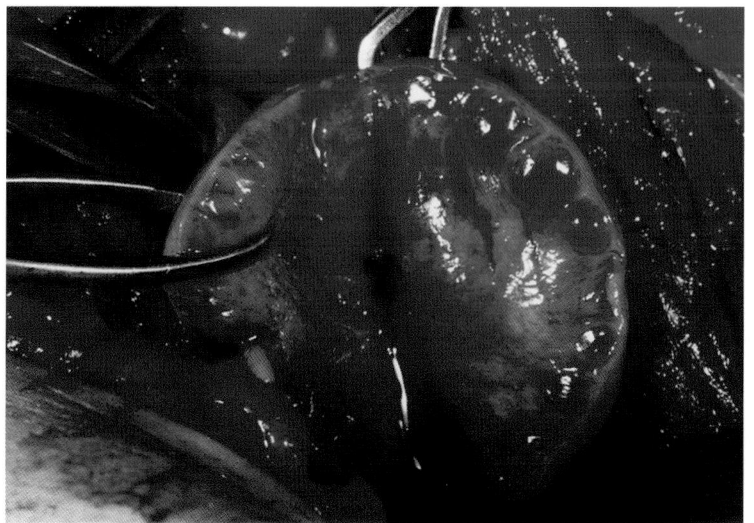

Fig. 91 Cut surface of polycystic ovary.

Differential diagnosis

Increased adrenal androgen production could also mean:

- Cushing syndrome
- adrenal hyperplasia
- adrenal carcinoma

Hirsutism could also be familial, or due to drugs, while other causes of secondary amenorrhoea include hyperprolactinaemia. Other causes of infertility can be found on page 64.

Investigation

Biochemical Serum LH, FSH, prolactin, testosterone (DHEAS, androstenedione).

Ultrasound Ovaries and pelvis (Fig. 92) (laparoscopy).

Management

Hirsutism Management includes:

- cosmetic treatments (cream, waxing and electrolysis)
- oral contraceptive pill with low androgenic progestogen
- anti-androgens (cyproterone acetate) and spironolactone

Obesity is treated with diet ± metformin.

Oligoamenorrhoea/amenorrhoea Treatment includes:

- oral contraceptive pill to produce regular withdrawal bleeds
- clomiphene (will produce regular cycles in 50% but will also induce ovulation)

Infertility Induction of ovulation with clomiphene is successful in 70–80% of women with PCOS, with pregnancy rates equivalent to regularly ovulating women. If not successful, HMG, with or without pituitary downregulation using LHRH analogues, is usually effective. This latter regime can result in severe ovarian hyperstimulation (Fig. 93).

Complications

This group of obese, anovulatory women are more likely to develop endometrial hyperplasia and adenocarcinoma in later life. Regular shedding of the endometrium induced by progestogens or the oral contraceptive pill seems a logical, though unproven, prophylaxis.

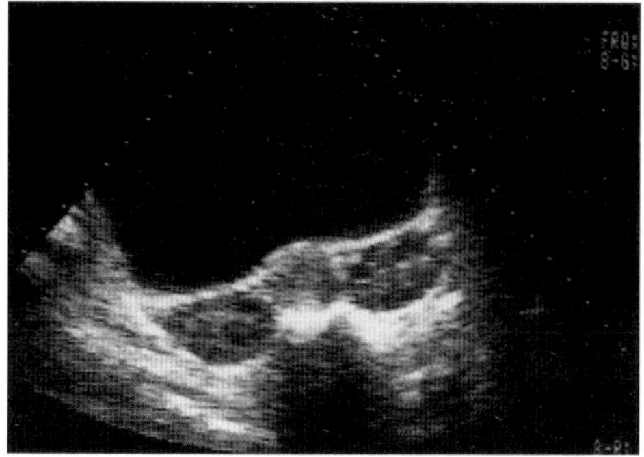

Fig. 92 Ultrasound showing polycystic ovaries.

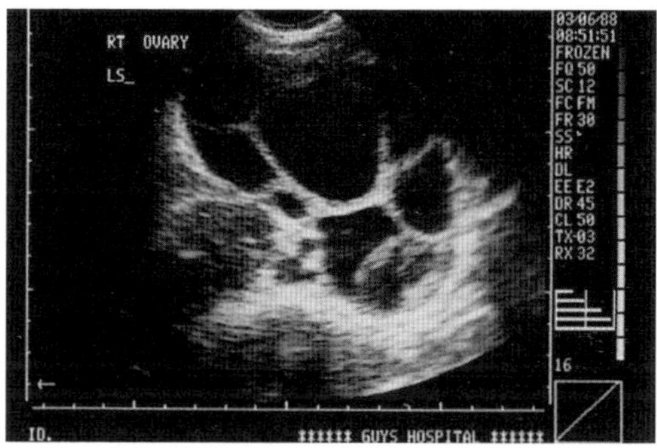

Fig. 93 Hyperstimulation in a polycystic ovary as seen by ultrasound.

12 Benign and malignant conditions of the vulva and vagina

Pruritus vulvae

Aetiology

Vulval irritation can occur at any age, and the causes are numerous. The most common are infection, oestrogen deficiency and vulval dermatoses in the older woman.

Pathology

The most common infective agent is *Candida*. Non-infectious causes include lichen sclerosus (Fig. 94), Paget's disease and vulval intraepithelial neoplasia (VIN). Paget's disease of the vulva usually presents in the elderly (Fig. 95). VIN is a precursor of invasive carcinoma.

Clinical features

Irritation and itchiness of the vulva are present. On examination there may be evidence of excoriation, discoloration (Fig. 94), thickening or thinning of the vulval skin.

Bartholin's glands

These are paired structures that lie deep to the posterior introitus. They can become infected and present as a large, tender, swollen abscess. Marsupialization is the treatment of choice. Cyst formation can also occur (Fig. 96).

Urethral caruncle

The external urethral meatus protrudes (Fig. 97) and swells. It may bleed, and may be very tender. Urethral caruncles are often associated with infection. If surgery is performed, the excised piece of tissue should be sent for histological confirmation to exclude urethral carcinoma.

Condylomata acuminata

Venereal warts are common on the vulva (Fig. 66) or in the vagina. They can be treated by topical applications, local destructive methods or surgery.

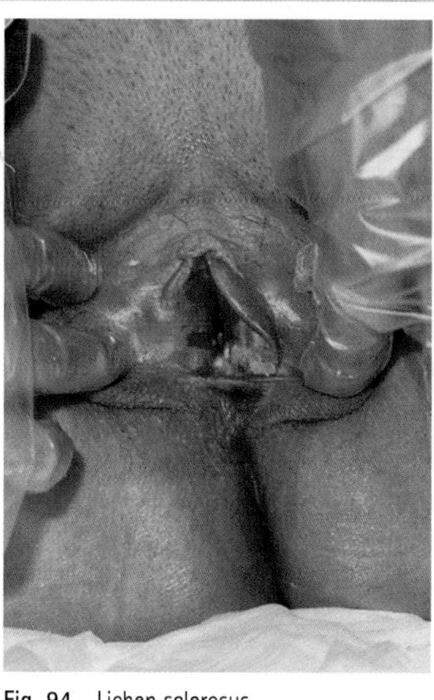

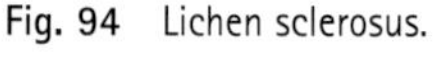

Fig. 94 Lichen sclerosus.

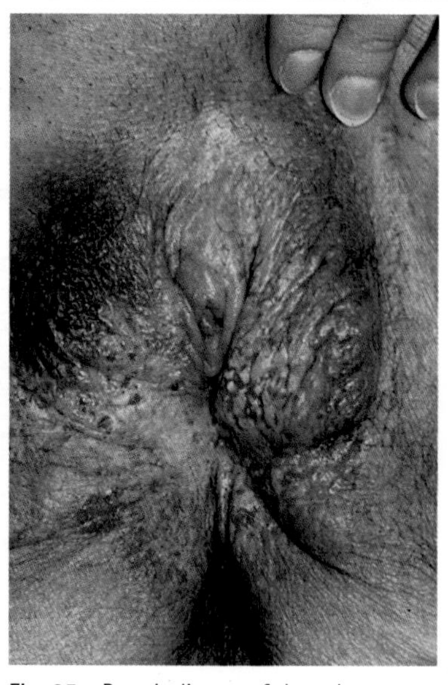

Fig. 95 Paget's disease of the vulva.

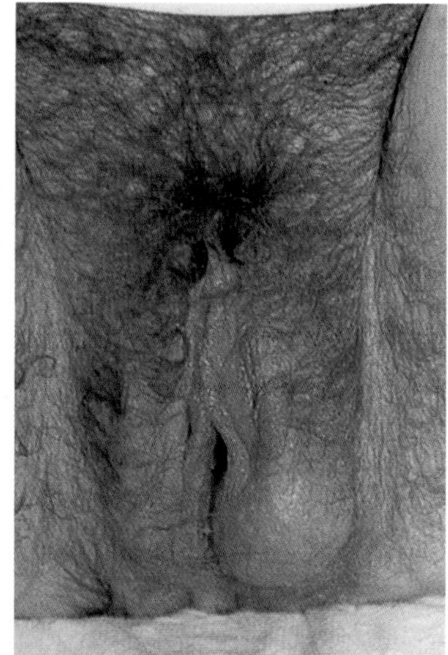

Fig. 96 Bartholin's cyst.

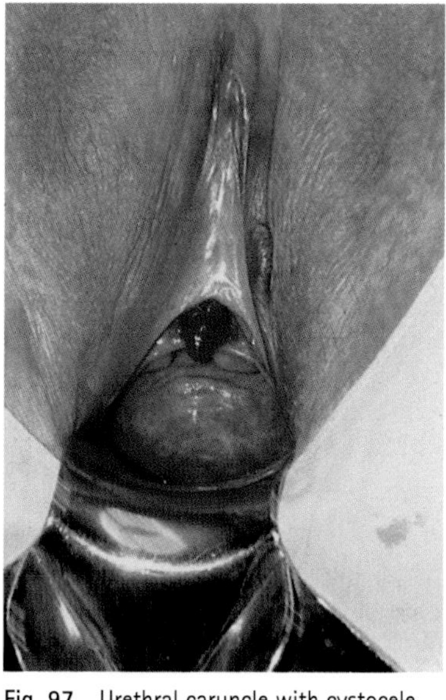

Fig. 97 Urethral caruncle with cystocele.

Cancer of the vulva

Incidence and aetiology

Vulval carcinoma is an uncommon condition usually confined to older women and associated with underlying vulval conditions such as lichen sclerosus et atrophicus. There has, however, been a rise in incidence in younger women, associated with high-risk HPV types and smoking.

Pathology

Carcinoma of the vulva (Fig. 98) is usually slow-growing and the vast majority are squamous cell tumours. Most of the lymphatics drain directly to the superficial and deep inguinal nodes and then to the iliac chain. Basal cell carcinoma and melanoma are rare.

Clinical features

Usually presents with a lump or mass or ulceration and a history of pruritus.

Management

All suspicious lesions must be biopsied. If vulval intra-epithelial neoplasia is diagnosed, excision may be appropriate. Invasive carcinoma is best managed by radical excision of the tumour (Figs 99, 100, 101), i.e. achieving deep clearance down to the underlying fascia, and an adequate skin margin of >1 cm. Removal of the inguinofemoral lymph nodes is necessary if the depth of invasion of the tumour is >1 mm. If the tumour is well lateralized only the nodes on that side need be removed. If the tumour is central, bilateral inguinofemoral lymphadenectomy is indicated.

Chemo-irradiation is used as first-line treatment if the tumour is not excisable and radiotherapy is sometimes necessary if the tumour extends close to the excision margins.

Complications

Complications include wound haematoma and lymphocele formation at the groin as a consequence of node dissection; these usually resolve with intermittent drainage. Lymphoedema can be a chronic complication.

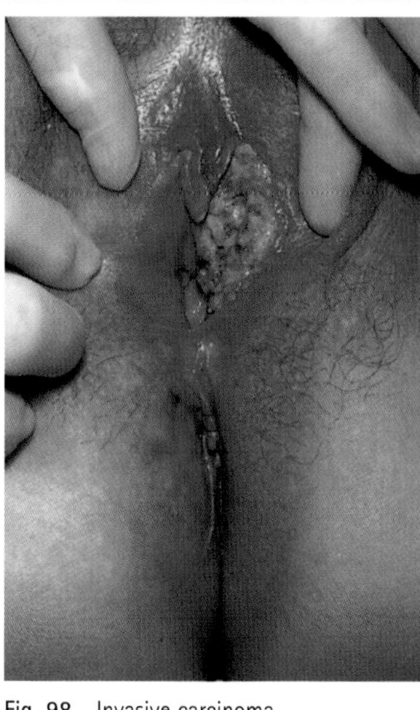

Fig. 98 Invasive carcinoma.

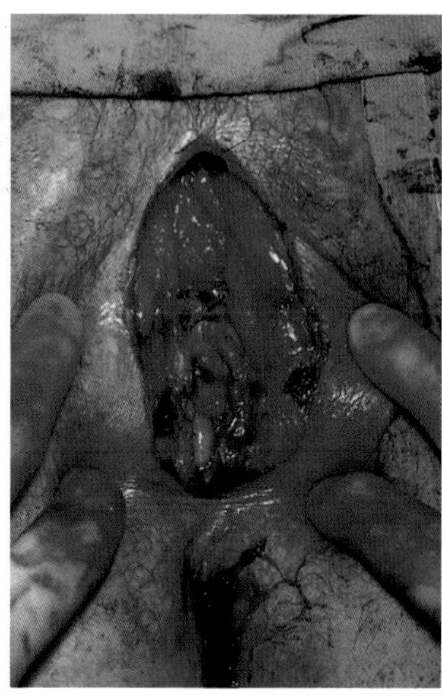

Fig. 99 Excision of the vulva.

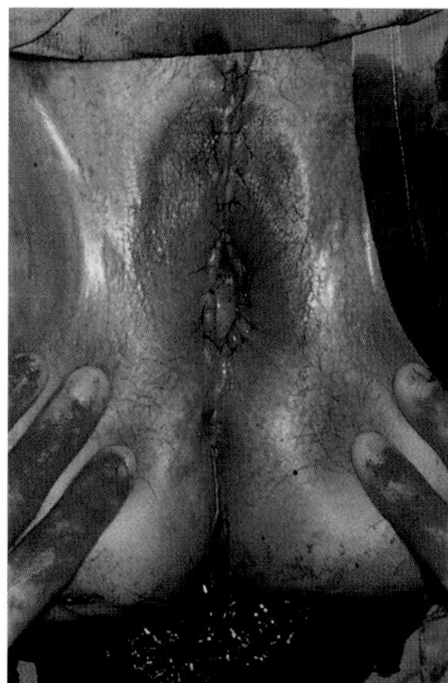

Fig. 100 Postoperative appearance.

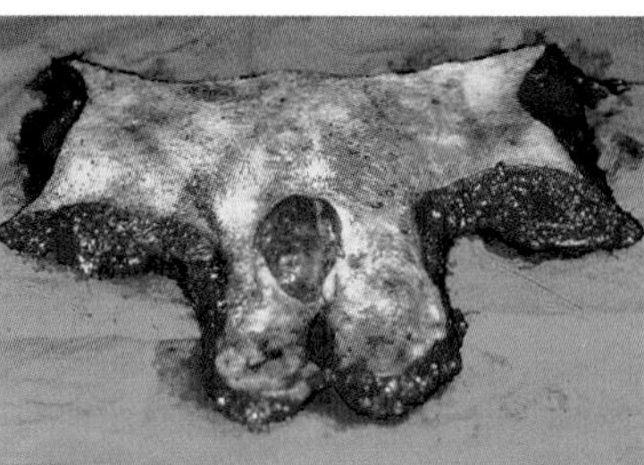

Fig. 101 Surgical specimen of vulval carcinoma.

13 Benign, premalignant and malignant conditions of the vagina and cervix

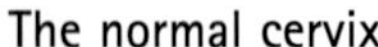

The normal cervix

The normal ectocervix is covered with stratified squamous epithelium (Fig. 102). The endocervical canal is lined by columnar epithelium (Fig. 103). The junction between these two types is known as the *squamocolumnar junction.*

The position of the squamocolumnar junction varies. Puberty, pregnancy and the use of the oral contraceptive pill cause eversion of the canal, thus displaying a greater area of columnar epithelium, which has a red appearance to the naked eye. This is termed *ectopy.*

The area medial to the original squamocolumnar junction is termed the transformation zone. It is in this area that metaplasia (the change of one cell type to another) takes place, i.e. columnar cells are transformed to mature squamous epithelium.

Benign conditions

Cervicitis

Certain bacteria preferentially infect columnar epithelium, e.g. *Chlamydia trachomatis* and *Neisseria gonorrhoeae*, giving rise to appearances described as cervicitis.

Cervical fibroids

These may be pedunculated or within the body of the cervix, perhaps growing to a size that fills the vagina.

Cervical polyps

These usually arise from the endocervix and are pedunculated with a covering of endocervical epithelium. They vary considerably in size and appear as bright red vascular growths (Fig. 104). Endocervical polyps may be symptomless or may present with irregular vaginal bleeding and/or postcoital bleeding. Treatment is by avulsion. If the base is broad it may require ligation.

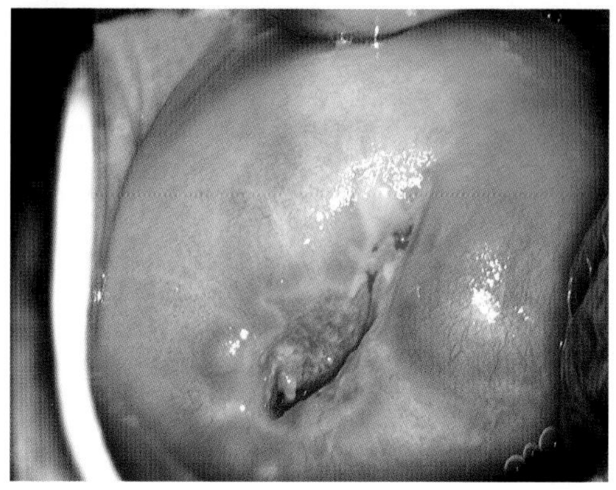

Fig. 102 Colpophotograph of a normal cervix.

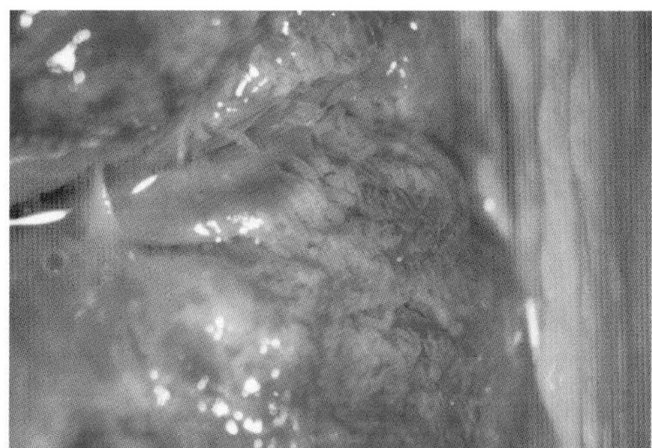

Fig. 103 Cervical columnar epithelium – high power.

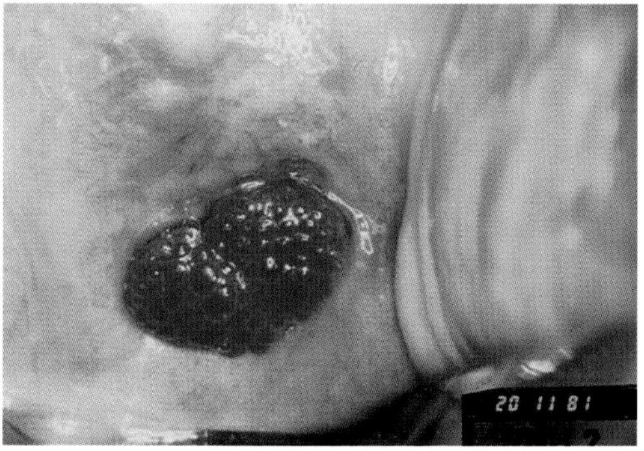

Fig. 104 Endocervical polyp – colpophotograph.

Premalignant conditions

In the transformation zone of the cervix there is an ongoing process of metaplasia (change of cell type from columnar to squamous epithelium). Interference with this normal process by factors such as wart virus (HPV) means that the resultant squamous cells are irregular (dysplastic).

Clinical features

Premalignant conditions of the cervix do not look abnormal to the naked eye. They are identified by cervical smear screening. The smear may demonstrate dyskaryotic cells (Fig. 105), graded as mild, moderate or severe (Fig. 106), depending on the degree of atypia. A dyskaryotic cell is clearly recognizable as a squamous cell but displays some of the features of malignancy: the nucleus is enlarged, the chromatin is increased and the nuclear borders are irregular.

Investigations

Women should have smears taken at 3-yearly intervals. Women should be referred for colposcopy after two borderline or visibly dyskaryotic smears, or one moderate or severely dyskaryotic smear.

Colposcopy is used to identify the lesion giving rise to the dyskaryotic cells exfoliated by the cervical smear. Using acetic acid to stain the cervix, areas of immature metaplasia and dysplasia (Fig. 107) are seen as white ('acetowhite'). The density of this whiteness together with other features, including *punctation* (Fig. 108), *mosaicism* (Fig. 109, p. 83), and *atypical vessel formation,* suggest the degree of abnormality present. The abnormal areas can be biopsied or excised to make a histological diagnosis.

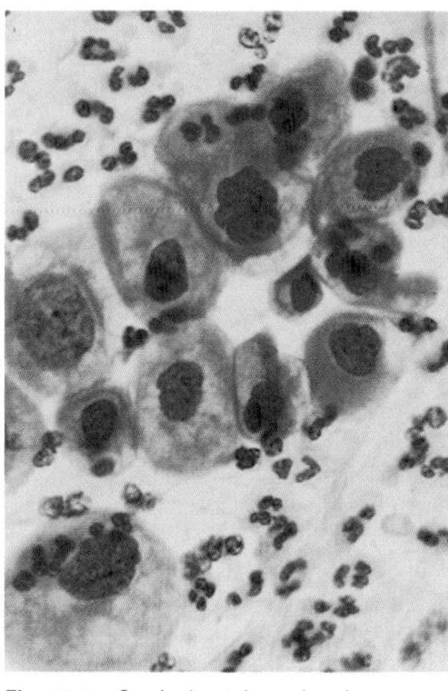

Fig. 105 Cervical cytology showing dyskaryosis.

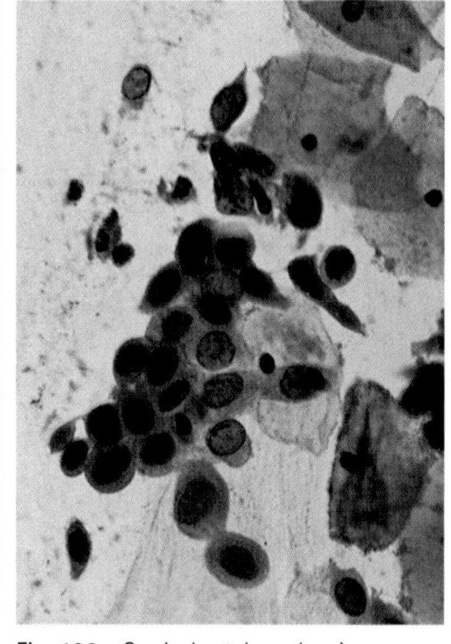

Fig. 106 Cervical cytology showing severe dyskaryosis.

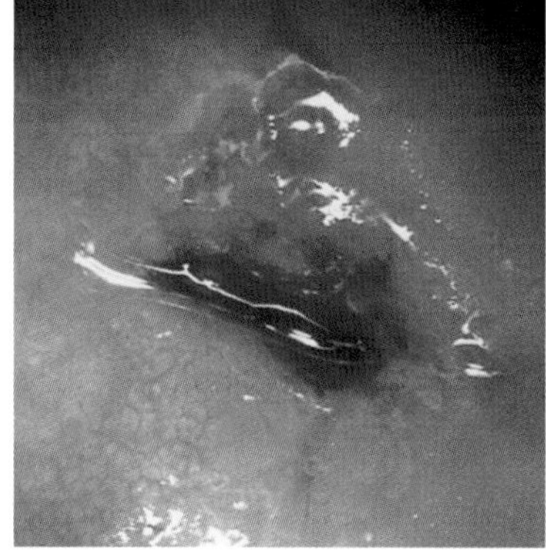

Fig. 107 Acetowhite changes.

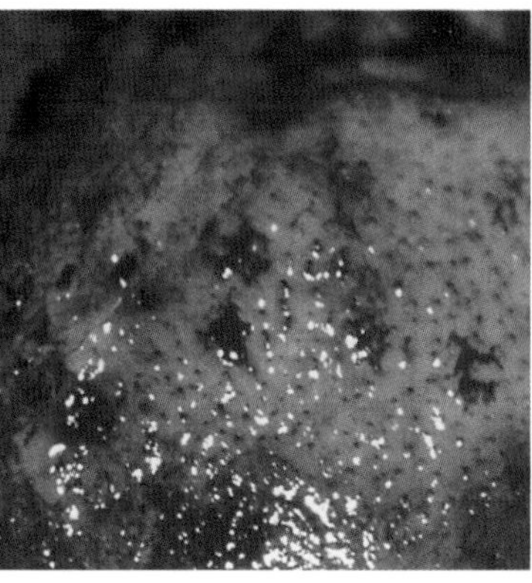

Fig. 108 Marked punctation.

Grading

The histological findings are graded as CIN (cervical intraepithelial neoplasia) I, II and III, depending on the degree of dysplasia. Dysplasia is a histological term used to describe a lesion in which part of the thickness of the epithelium is replaced by atypical cells (Fig. 110).

If untreated, CIN may progress to cervical cancer.

- *CIN I*: the atypia is confined to the basal one-third of the epithelium.
- *CIN II*: the basal two-thirds are involved and the changes are more marked.
- *CIN III*: nuclear abnormalities are present throughout the whole thickness of the epithelium (Figs 111, 112).

Predisposing factors

High-risk HPV types, i.e. 16, 18 and 32, and smoking are the major factors currently associated with CIN.

Management

CIN can be managed conservatively with regular follow-up until the abnormality regresses.

CIN II and III are usually treated by loop excision. This can be performed under local anaesthetic and as it provides a good histopathology specimen, can be done at the first visit (see and treat). Laser ablation and electrical cauterization can be used once a biopsy specimen has been obtained. Cone biopsy is necessary if the upper limit of the transformation zone cannot be visualized in the canal.

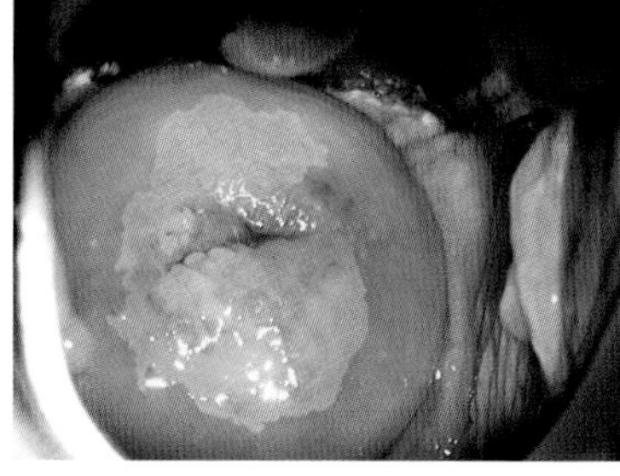

Fig. 109 Florid mosaicism.

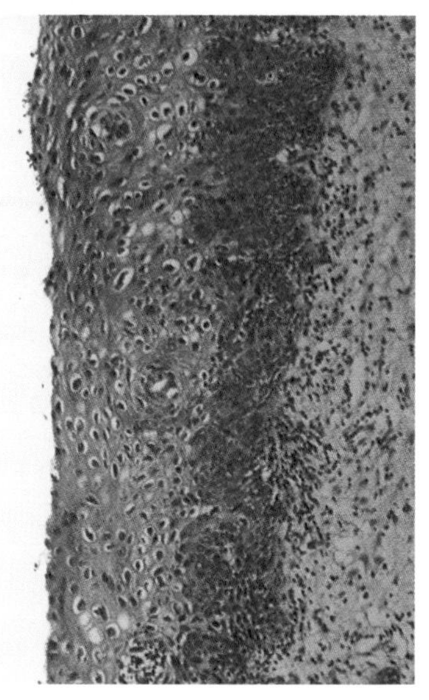

Fig. 110 Human papilloma virus and CIN.

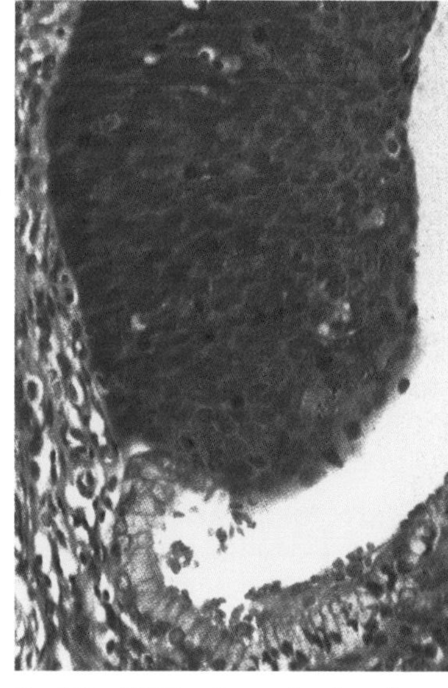

Fig. 111 CIN III and normal endocervix.

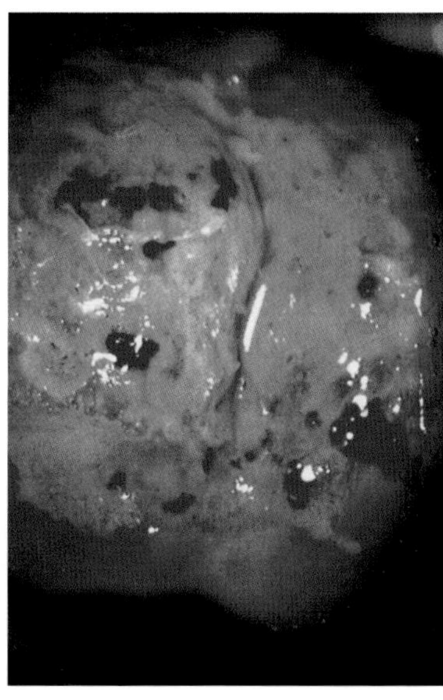

Fig. 112 Macroscopic view of CIN III.

Carcinoma of the cervix

Incidence

In England and Wales there are currently 2700 cases of cervical cancer per year and 1200 deaths from the disease. Incidence and mortality are falling because of the effectiveness of the NHS cervical screening programme in the UK.

Aetiology

Carcinoma of the cervix is more frequently seen in developing countries and its incidence is higher in lower socioeconomic groups. Cancer of the cervix is essentially a sexually transmitted disease.

A number of factors may predispose to cervical cancer. Presently the wart virus has the strongest association. Smoking may also have a role.

Staging

Cancer of the cervix is staged clinically (by examination under anaesthesia, cervical biopsy, hysteroscopy and cystoscopy) because worldwide most patients will be treated only with radiotherapy. In developed countries MRI scanning is used increasingly as a staging tool.

Stage I

- 1a: Stromal invasion of ≤5 mm, extension ≤5 mm with lateral extension of ≤7 mm
- 1b: Clinically visible lesions limited to the cervix –
  1b1 ≤4 cm
  1b2 >4 cm

Stage II

The carcinoma extends beyond the cervix but has not extended onto the pelvic side wall. The carcinoma involves the vagina but not as far as the lower one-third.

Stage III

Carcinoma extends to the pelvic side wall. The lower one-third of the vagina may be involved. All cases with a hydronephrosis or a non-functioning kidney, unless they are known to be due to another cause.

Stage IV

Carcinoma has extended beyond the true pelvis or has clinically involved the mucosa of the bladder or rectum (Fig. 114).

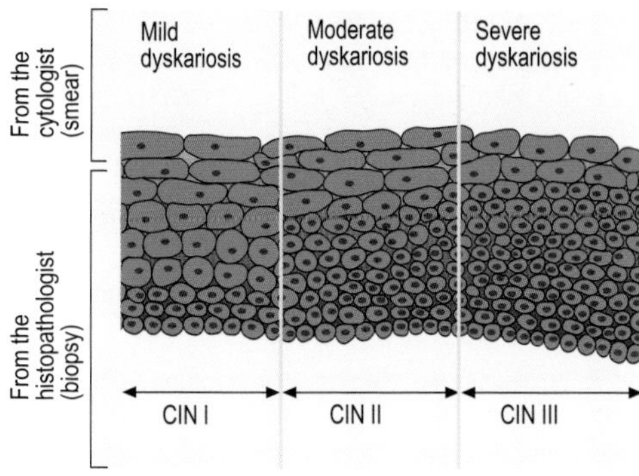

Fig. 113 The CIN grading system.

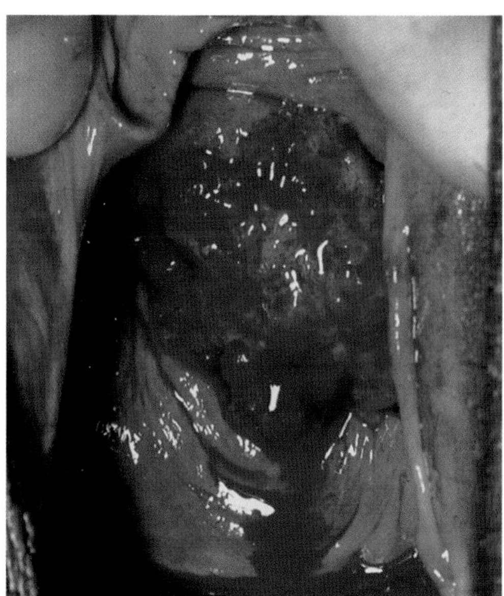

Fig. 114 Frank invasive carcinoma of the cervix.

Pathology

Up to 90% of cervical cancers are squamous cell tumours originating in the transformation zone. Adenocarcinomas account for the remainder of cases. Cervical cancer spreads by direct extension or via the lymphatics.

Clinical features

Patients may present with vaginal bleeding, particularly after intercourse. There may be vaginal discharge. Early lesions may be symptomless and are detected by screening.

Investigations

Once the diagnosis is confirmed histologically an EUA is necessary for staging. Chest X-ray, IVP and routine biochemical and haematological investigations are usually required. CT scan is helpful in advanced and recurrent disease.

Management

Hysterectomy is usually advised for microinvasive disease. Cone biopsy may be considered in a young woman desiring children. Stage Ib or IIa cervical cancer can be treated by either radiotherapy or radical Wertheim's hysterectomy (removal of the uterus, fallopian tubes, upper one-third of the vagina, parametrium and pelvic lymph nodes). Wertheim's hysterectomy is the treatment of choice in younger women who wish to retain ovarian function and avoid vaginal stenosis and gastrointestinal side effects, which may be caused by radiotherapy. Radical trachelectomy (the removal of the cervix but not the uterine body – Fig. 115) is being evaluated as a fertility-sparing treatment for some women with early-stage disease. The results of radiotherapy and radical surgery in early stage disease are similar, both having 5-year survival rates in excess of 80%. The finding of tumour in lymph nodes will halve this survival rate. Radiotherapy is commonly used in more advanced diseases in combination with platinum-based chemotherapy.

Carcinoma of the vagina

Rare and tends to occur mainly in the 6th and 7th decades. Presenting symptoms are vaginal bleeding or a purulent discharge. Treatment of the condition is determined by histology, staging and the health of the patient. Surgery, radiotherapy and a combination of both have been used.

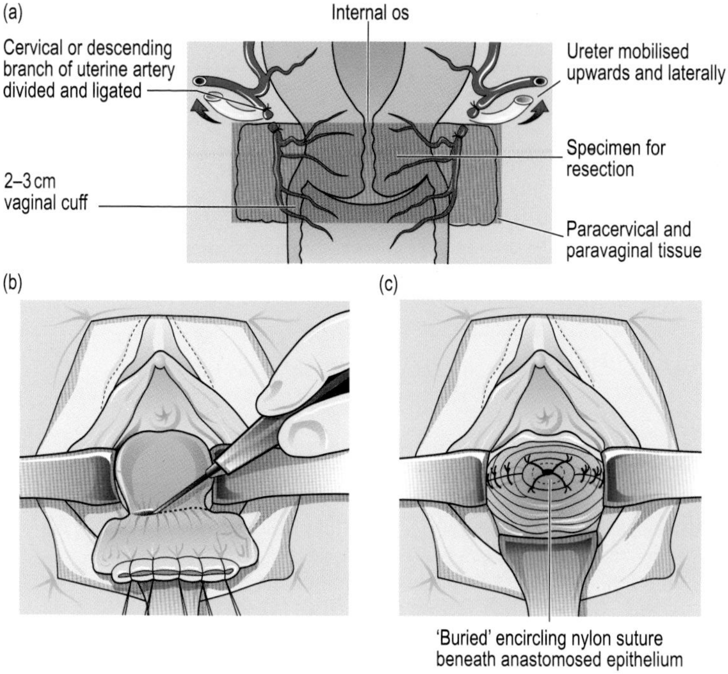

(a)
Internal os
Cervical or descending branch of uterine artery divided and ligated
Ureter mobilised upwards and laterally
Specimen for resection
2–3 cm vaginal cuff
Paracervical and paravaginal tissue

(b)

(c)

'Buried' encircling nylon suture beneath anastomosed epithelium

Fig. 115 Radical trachelectomy.

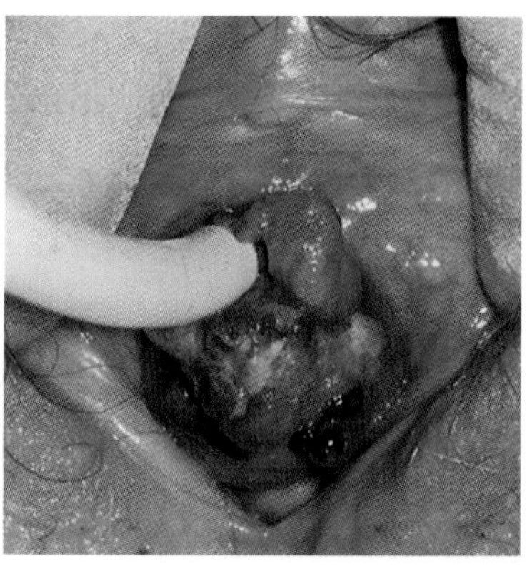

Fig. 116 Vaginal carcinoma.

14 Benign and malignant conditions of the uterus

Congenital anomalies

Congenital absence of the uterus is rare, and in such cases a rudimentary vagina may be present. Congenital anomalies range from an arcuate uterus to a complete duplication of the uterus and cervix (Figs 117, 118).

Fibroids

Definition

Common smooth muscle tumours also known as leiomyomata. Aetiology unknown.

Incidence

Fibroids occur in more than 20% of Caucasian women over 30 years.

Classification

- *Subserous:* project from the peritoneal surface of the uterus
- *Intramural:* lie within the uterine wall
- *Submucous:* encroach on the uterine cavity
- *Pedunculated:* can arise from subserous or submucous

Pathology

Fibroids arise from smooth muscle cells during reproductive life and can increase in size in response to oestrogen.

Clinical features

The majority of fibroids are symptomless. They may cause menorrhagia, abdominal distension and pressure symptoms such as urinary frequency. Pain is unusual unless there is red degeneration or torsion of a pedunculated fibroid.

Abdominal examination may reveal a palpable mass arising from the pelvis. Pelvic examination will confirm this and the outline may be irregular.

Investigations

These include ultrasonography, EUA, hysteroscopy and endometrial biopsy if abnormal bleeding.

Management

Treatment can either be conservative or surgical (Fig. 119).

Complications

The poor vascularity of fibroids encourages degeneration (hyaline, cystic, red, sarcomatous), calcification (Fig. 120) and/or necrosis. Fibroids can also become infected, tort and rarely metastasize.

Fig. 117 Laparoscopic view of bicornuate uterus.

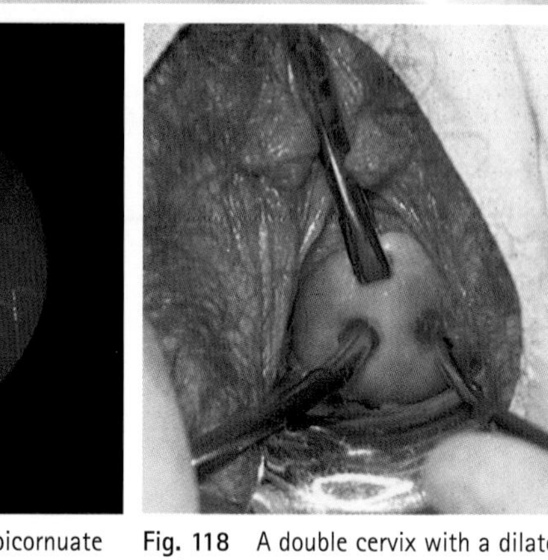

Fig. 118 A double cervix with a dilator in each os.

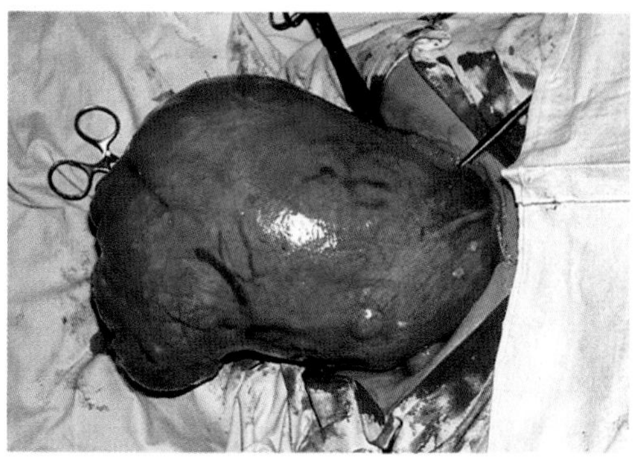

Fig. 119 Enlarged fibroid uterus – operative specimen.

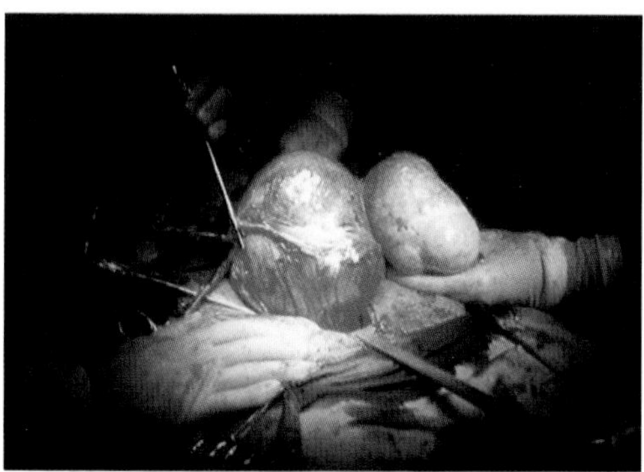

Fig. 120 Enlarged uterus with a pedunculated fibroid arising from the left lateral fundus.

Uterine cancer

Classification

The majority of lesions are adenocarcinoma (Fig. 121), and the staging is as follows:

Stage I: confined to the body of the uterus.
Stage II: involves the body and the cervix.
Stage III: extends beyond uterus but not beyond the true pelvis.
Stage IV: extends outside true pelvis or involves bladder or rectum.

Aetiology

Endometrial cancer occurs mostly in postmenopausal women and women who have had prolonged exposure to oestrogen stimulation, i.e. nulliparous women, late menopause, obese women and women with polycystic ovaries. Hyperplasia is a precursor.

Clinical features

Postmenopausal bleeding is the classic presentation for endometrial carcinoma and therefore requires investigation. It is rare in women under the age of 40, unless there are predisposing factors, e.g. PCO.

Clinical features

Abdominal and pelvic examinations, including a cervical smear, should be carried out in all cases. Transvaginal ultrasound scanning may be helpful in identifying changes (>5 mm endometrial thickening is suspicious). Endometrial sampling and/or hysteroscopy (Fig. 122) can be performed in the outpatient clinic or, if that is not possible, under general anaesthetic.

Investigations

A total abdominal hysterectomy and bilateral salpingo-oophorectomy is performed during a staging operation which involves taking peritoneal washings. The role of lymphadenectomy in endometrial cancer is under evaluation. Adjuvant radiotherapy is sometimes used for high-grade lesions and cancers that involve the outer half of the endometrium to reduce the risk of local or regional recurrence.

Management

Factors influencing survival endometrial carcinoma are age at diagnosis, stage of disease, pathological type and degree of differentiation of the lesion and the depth of myometrial invasion.

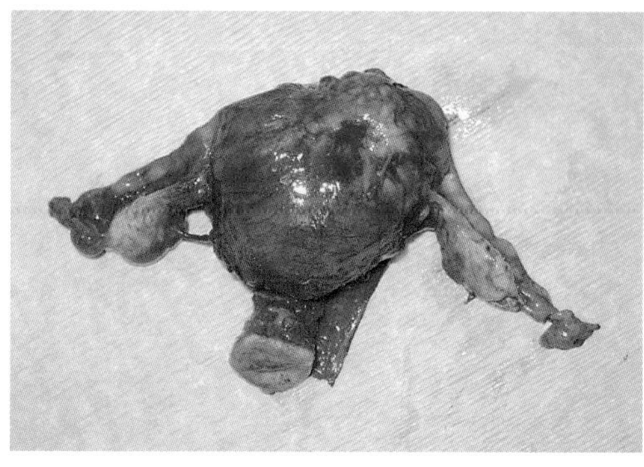

Fig. 121 Surgical specimen of an endometrial cancer spreading through the serosa.

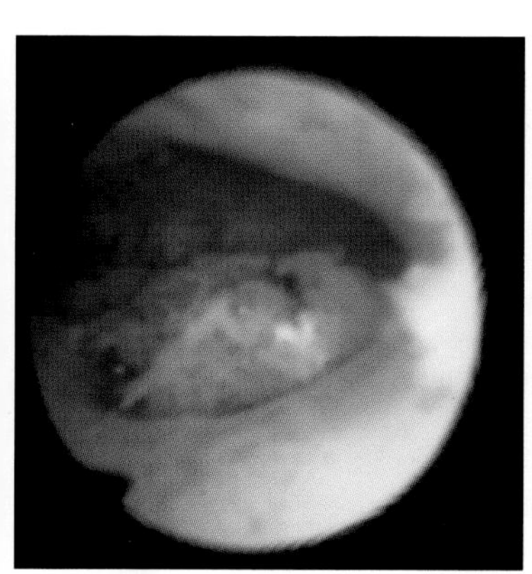

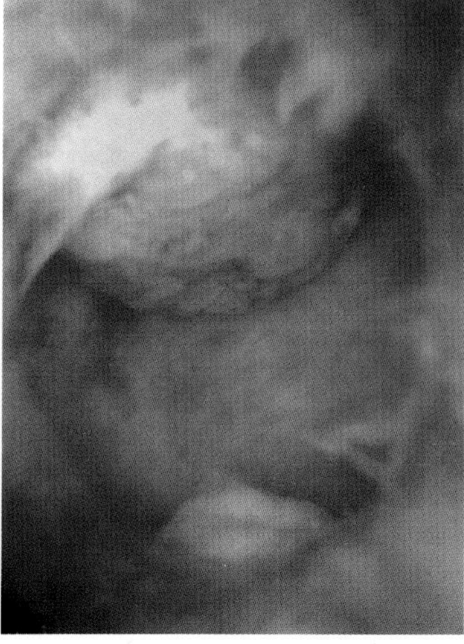

Fig. 122a&b Hysteroscopic views of endometrial carcinoma.

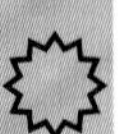

15 Benign and malignant conditions of the fallopian tubes

The fimbriae of the fallopian tubes pick up the ovum after it is released from the follicle and the cilia of the endosalpinx transport it to the site of fertilization. Sperm are carried there by the cilia from the uterine end of the tube.

Tubal infection

The tubes can become blocked by infection (or inflammation following trauma). The result of this can be tubal abscess or hydrosalpinx (Fig. 123).

Clinical features

Tubal infection may present with pain of an acute abdomen, especially if an abscess has formed. A hydrosalpinx may be symptomless.

Investigations

Laparoscopy is useful for inspection of the peritoneal aspect of the tubes. Exudate may be seen over the tubes, especially at the fimbriae. If the fimbriae are clubbed, this indicates chronic damage. Fresh and old adhesions may be seen. A hydrosalpinx will be visualized as a swollen tube but not actively infected. In the absence of acute infection, dye can be injected through the cervix. If there is no tubal blockage, filling of the tubes and free spill into the peritoneal cavity can be seen. Hysterosalpingography is a useful investigative technique.

Management

Acute infection should be treated appropriately. Infertility due to tubal damage can be treated by tubal surgery or in vitro fertilization to overcome tubal blockage.

Cancer of the fallopian tube

Primary cancer of the fallopian tube (Fig. 124) is rare; secondary disease from adjacent structures is more common. The symptoms are classically a watery, bloody vaginal discharge. On examination, an adnexal mass may be felt. The ovarian tumour marker CA125 is often raised. The treatment is total abdominal hysterectomy and bilateral oophorectomy followed by chemotherapy as for ovarian cancer.

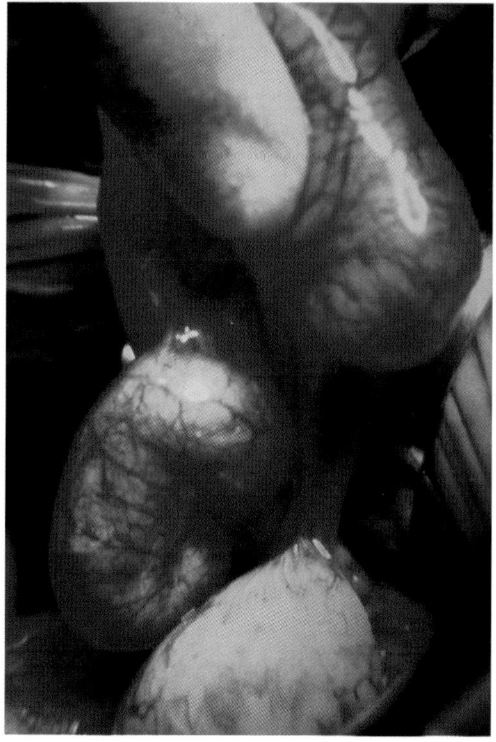

Fig. 123 Hydrosalpinx.

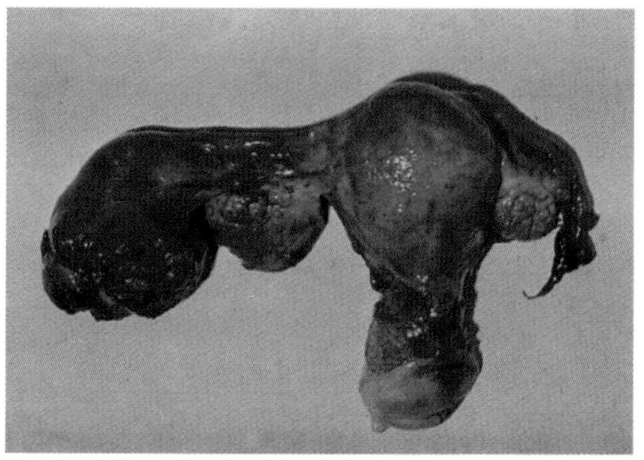

Fig. 124 Carcinoma of the fallopian tube.

16 Benign and malignant conditions of the ovary

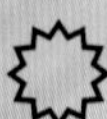

Ovarian cysts may be physiological, benign (Fig. 125) or malignant tumours. Ovarian pathology may give rise to symptoms:

- when ovarian enlargement causes pressure on the bladder or rectum or abdominal distension
- if the ovary/cyst torts, bleeds or ruptures
- should hormonal production be affected

Physiological cysts (distension cysts)

Clinical types

Follicular cysts Due to enlargement of follicles which fail to rupture. They may be associated with anovulatory cycles, fertility drugs and PCOs. Usually symptomless and resolve spontaneously.

Corpus luteum cysts Can cause amenorrhoea followed by heavy vaginal bleeding. Spontaneous resolution is the norm but intra-abdominal bleeding may cause significant pain.

Endometriomas Result from invagination of endometrial deposits on the surface of the ovary.

Polycystic ovaries Enlarged (Fig. 126), with numerous small subcapsular follicular cysts.

Ovarian tumours – benign and malignant

Incidence

Benign tumours of the ovary are common. Ovarian cancer has an incidence of 14:100 000 women in the UK. The incidence of ovarian cancer increases with age, with the peak incidence in the sixties.

Clinical features

Ovarian cancer is often either symptomless or associated with non-specific symptoms such as dyspepsia. A malignant tumour should be suspected in older women, especially if it is fixed, bilateral, rapid-growing or associated with ascites. A solid, or a mixed cystic and solid appearance on ultrasound scanning is also suggestive. In advanced disease there may be venous obstruction of the legs, pain and palpable supraclavicular lymphadenopathy.

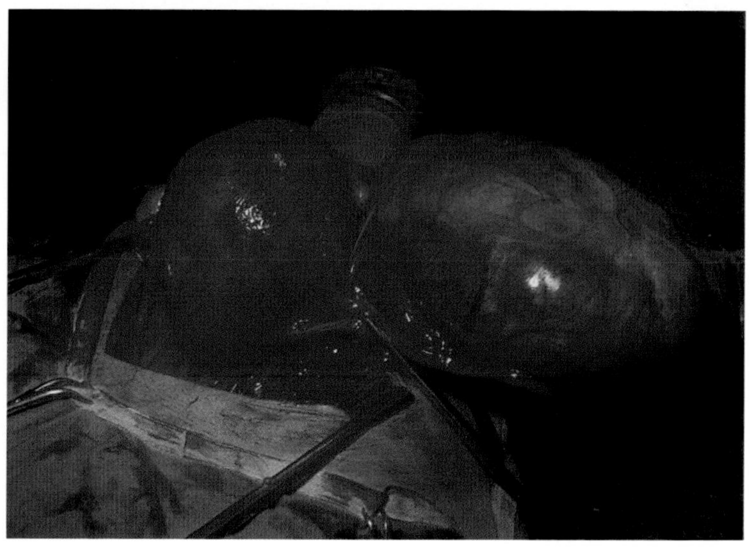

Fig. 125 Large benign ovarian cyst.

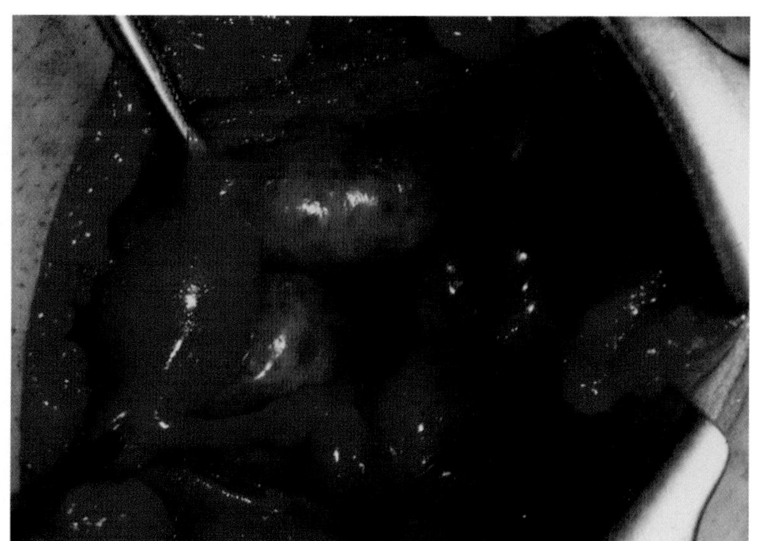

Fig. 126 'Kissing' polycystic ovaries.

Classification

Ovarian tumours can be derived from the following cell types:

- surface epithelium
- germ cells
- gonadal stroma

Secondary deposits from primary tumours of the breast, stomach, large bowel and uterus may also occur in the ovaries (Krukenberg tumours; Fig. 127).

Tumours derived from surface epithelium

About 90% of ovarian tumours originate from the surface epithelium. These are further subdivided into:

- *Serous*, e.g. serous cystadenoma (benign), serous cystadenocarcinoma (malignant, Fig. 128)
- *Mucinous*, e.g. mucinous cystadenoma, mucinous cystadenocarcinoma
- *Endometrioid*
- *Brenner tumours*
- *Clear cell tumours*

Epithelial ovarian tumours can be benign, of borderline malignancy, or frankly malignant. The malignant forms are collectively known as adenocarcinoma of the ovary.

Tumours derived from germ cells

The germ cells of the ovary are totipotent (i.e. can give rise to various types of tissues). Tumours of germ cells can contain a variety of tissues including teeth, bone, cartilage, muscle, thyroid and nervous tissue. The most common germ cell tumour is the benign cystic teratoma (dermoid cyst, Fig. 129). These are the most common tumours in young women. They are bilateral in 10–20% of cases.

Tumours derived from gonadal stroma

Sex cord tumours are rare. Granulosa cell tumours and thecomas secrete oestrogens and can therefore cause precocious puberty in premenarchal girls, and endometrial hyperplasia and postmenopausal bleeding in older women. More than 50% of granulosa cell tumours are malignant; the vast majority of thecomas are benign. Sertoli–Leydig tumours may secrete androgens and can therefore cause progressive virilization.

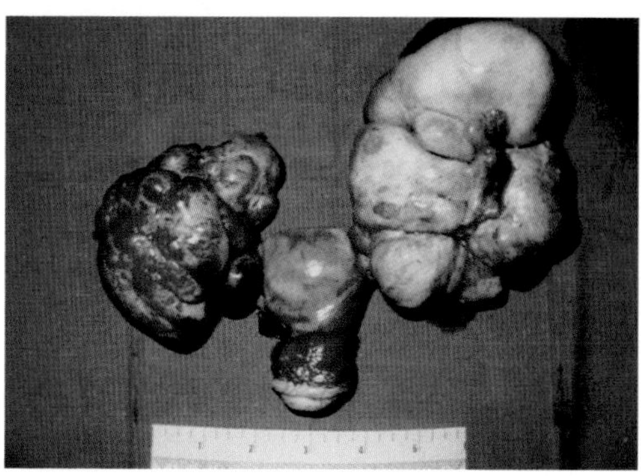

Fig. 127 Bilateral Krukenberg tumours.

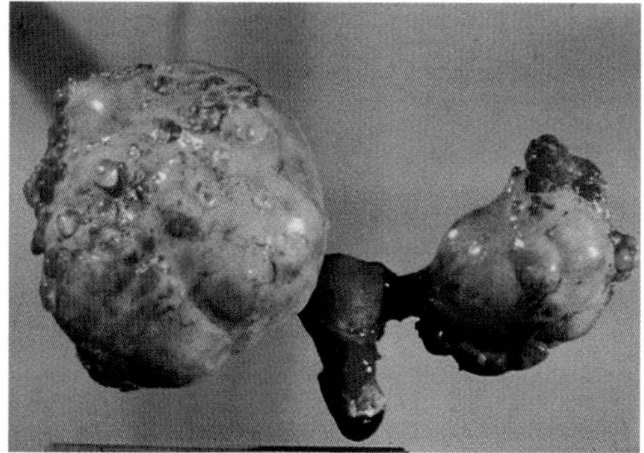

Fig. 128 Serous cystadenocarcinoma.

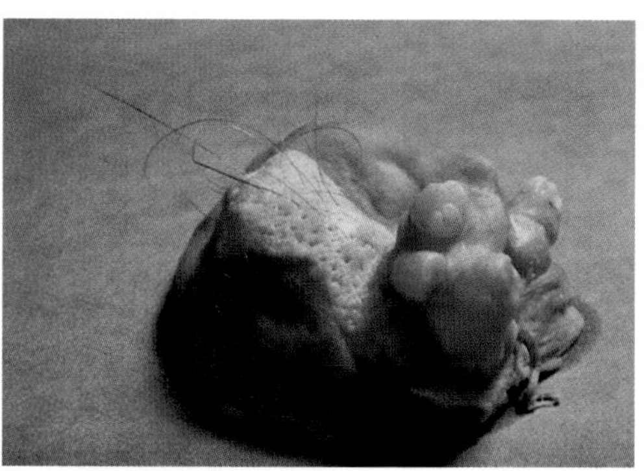

Fig. 129 Benign cystic teratoma.

Management

Before embarking upon surgery, the risk of malignancy must be assessed to prevent inexperienced operators encountering ovarian cancer (Figs 130, 131).

Ovarian cancer

An adequate preoperative assessment should be made, with a general examination including the breasts and lymph nodes. With preoperative ultrasound and measurement of the serum tumour marker CA125 to exclude/reduce the chances of malignancy, laparoscopic removal of the cyst/ovary is often employed. Laparotomy aims include: adequate staging and removal of all visible tumour deposits (Figs 132, 133).

Staging requires thorough inspection of the whole abdominal cavity through a vertical incision. Peritoneal washings are taken and the following are either removed or biopsied: parietal peritoneum, omentum, uterus and other ovary, bowel and mesentery, diaphragm, and pelvic and para-aortic lymph nodes.

Surgical measures

In most cases of ovarian cancer the aim is cystoreductive surgery followed by chemotherapy.

Prognosis

The 5-year survival rates for primary ovarian cancer are as follows: Ia 85%, Ib–IIa 40%, IIb 25%, IIc–III 15%, IV <5%. The prognosis has changed very little in the last 30 years because women continue to present late in the disease process.

Effective screening would be of value if it were possible to detect disease in its early stages, thus enabling more effective treatment. Ultrasound scanning and various tumour markers (e.g. CA 125) are currently used.

Screening or prophylactic removal of the ovaries may be appropriate for women at increased risk of ovarian cancer as demonstrated by a strong and reliable family history (e.g. two or more first-degree relatives with ovarian cancer) or a mutation of the *BRCA1* or *BRCA2* gene.

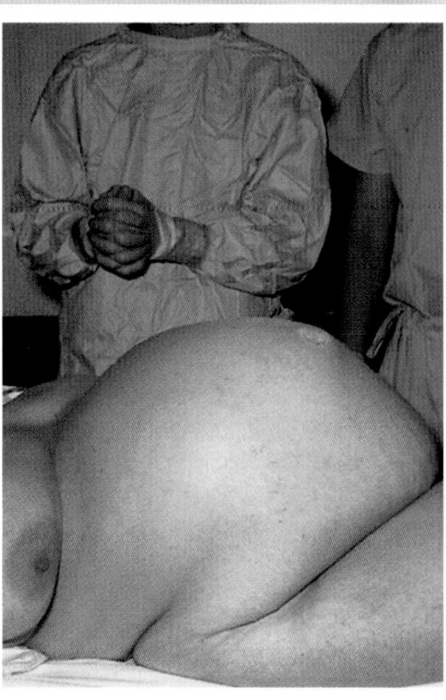

Fig. 130 Gross abdominal distension due to ovarian tumour.

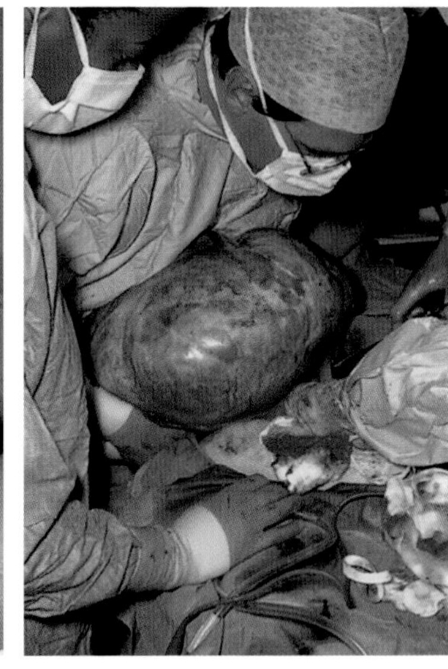

Fig. 131 Laparotomy findings in the case illustrated in Figure 130.

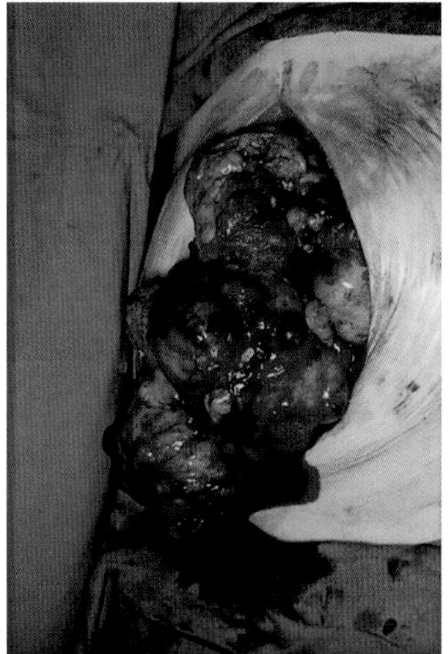

Fig. 132 Disseminated ovarian adenocarcinoma.

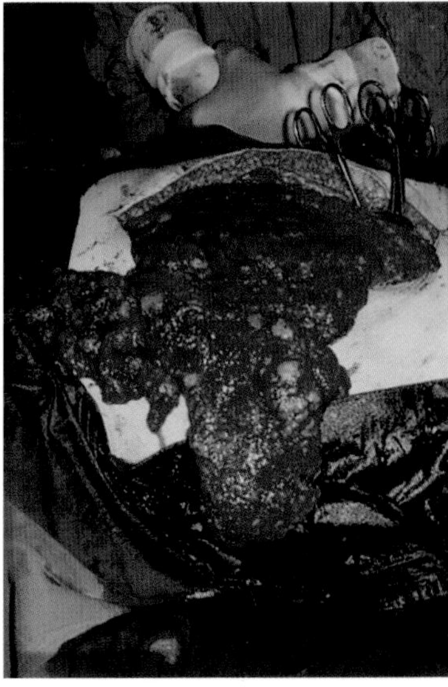

Fig. 133 Omental infiltration with ovarian adenocarcinoma.

The menopause and climacteric

Clinical features and pathology

Definition

The menopause is a woman's last menstrual period; the climacteric is the period of ovarian decline which includes the menopause.

Aetiology

At the beginning of the climacteric, the remaining ovarian follicles become increasingly resistant to gonadotrophin stimulation, and so more gonadotrophins are produced in response to the decreasing oestrogen levels.

Pathology

Atrophy occurs in all tissues that are sensitive to oestrogen, e.g. the urogenital system, breasts and skin.
Changes can also occur in bone. Osteoporosis is defined as a decreased amount of bony tissue per unit volume of bone, leading to structural weakness. With lowered oestrogen levels there appears to be a decrease in osteoblast function and an increase in bone resorption. This leads to a structural weakness in bone and increases the risk of fracture. The most common sites of fracture are the radius, the neck of the femur and the vertebral spine
(Fig. 134).
Cardiovascular disease also increases with the lowered oestrogen levels of the menopause. An increase in total cholesterol and low-density lipoprotein cholesterol occurs, along with a decline in high-density lipoprotein. While these lipid changes account for increased risk, other factors such as changes in glucose tolerance and the direct effects of oestrogen on arterial and venous blood flow are likely to be important.
Osteoporosis is described as the 'silent epidemic' in that the disease may not be detected until the woman falls and fractures her osteoporotic bone(s). Wedge fractures of the spine may be detected on X-ray (Fig. 135) and, if multiple, may produce the 'dowager's hump'.

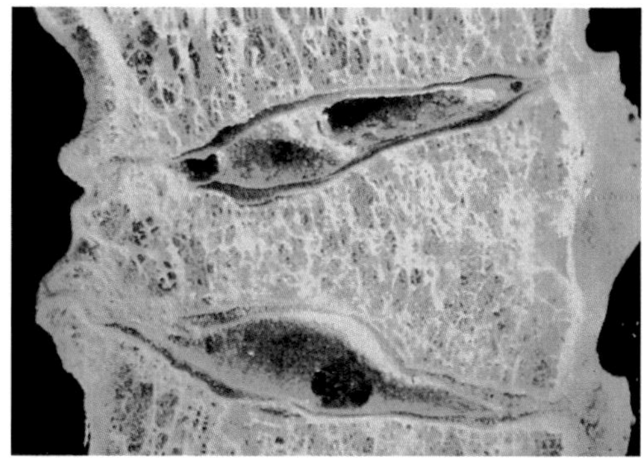

Fig. 134 Post-mortem specimen of osteoporotic wedge fracture.

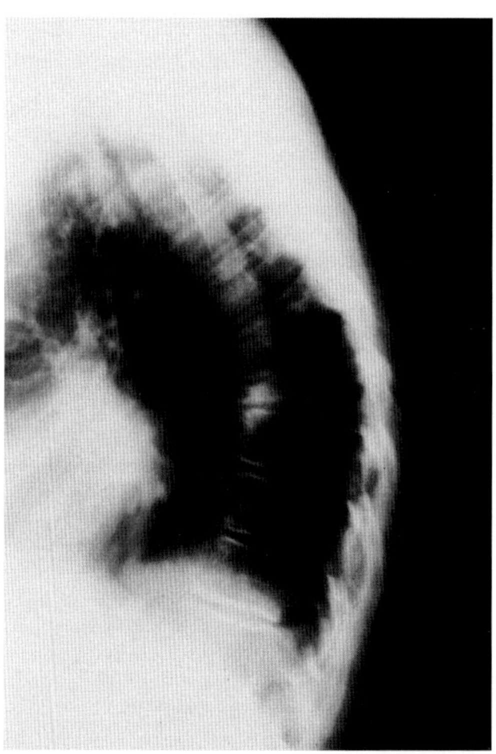

Fig. 135 X-ray showing wedge fracture of thoracic spine.

Clinical features

Hot flushes and night sweats are the classic symptoms of the menopause. Other symptoms include depression, vaginal soreness, vaginal dryness, urinary frequency, headaches and joint pains. On examination, hair loss, dry skin and vaginal atrophy may be present.

Investigations

If the diagnosis is in doubt, an FSH level of greater than 15 iu per litre will confirm ovarian failure.

Non-invasive methods are now available to assess bone density. Single photon absorptiometry was initially used, then dual photon, and now dual energy X-rays are used as the radioactive source (DXA, Fig. 136). Bone densitometry results of the hip are shown in Figure 137.

Blood pressure, breasts and cervical cytology should be checked as indicated. Mammography should be considered.

Management

Hormone replacement therapy is the most appropriate treatment for women with hypo-oestrogenic symptoms and for osteoporosis prevention.

There are various methods of administration (Fig. 138).

Oral Oestrogen tablets are given continuously and progestogen tablets are given for 12 days of each calendar month. For postmenopausal women (i.e. 1 year since LMP), continuous combined preparations of oestrogen and progestogen can be used to avoid monthly bleeding.

Parenteral Transdermal patches or oestrogen creams are available. Estradiol implants can be inserted subcutaneously every 6 months; a testosterone implant may be inserted at the same time if the woman is sexually active, to improve libido. Creams, pessaries or rings provide local treatment when used in the vagina.

With all the above preparations, progestogens must be given if there is a uterus.

Complications

HRT is associated with an increased risk of invasive breast carcinoma and venous thromboembolic disease.

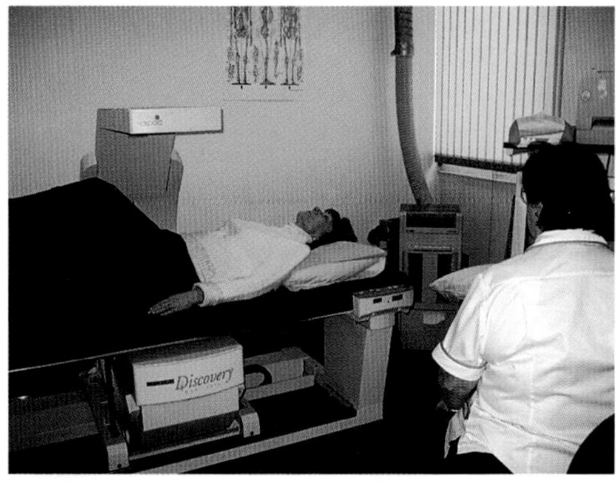

Fig. 136 Bone density measurement being performed.

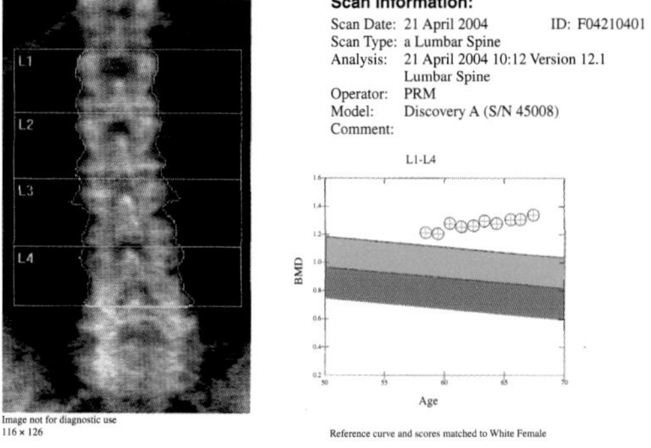

Fig. 137 DXA printout of bone density.

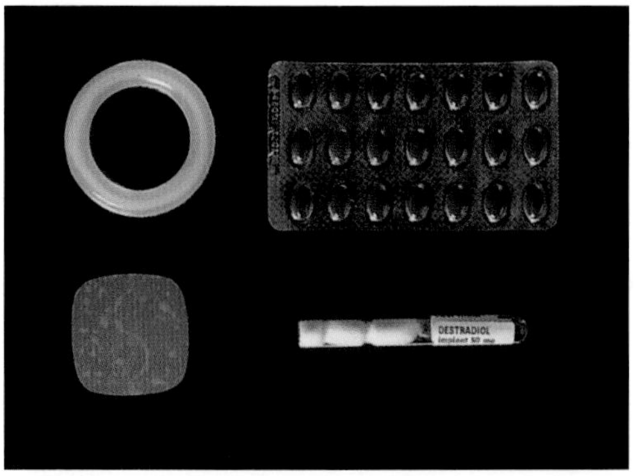

Fig. 138 HRT – implant, patch, oral tablets, vaginal ring.

18 Uterovaginal prolapse

Definition

The anterior vaginal wall is supported by the pubocervical fascia. This extends from the back of the symphysis pubis to the cervix and upper vagina. The posterior vaginal wall is supported by fibrous tissue of the rectovaginal septum and the levator ani muscles. The uterus is supported mainly by the cardinal or transverse cervical ligaments, which merge with the uterosacral ligaments before joining the cervix.

Uterovaginal prolapse is the downward displacement of the uterus (Fig. 139) and/or vagina towards or through the introitus. The bladder, urethra, rectum and bowel may also be involved.

Vaginal wall prolapse

A prolapse of the lowest one-third of the anterior vagina involves the urethra and is called a urethrocele. Prolapse of the upper two-thirds of the anterior vaginal wall involves the bladder and is therefore called a cystocele (Fig. 140). When the lower portion of the posterior vaginal wall prolapses, it brings with it the rectum and is therefore termed a rectocele. Prolapse of the vaginal wall above this involves the pouch of Douglas; it is called an enterocele (Fig. 141).

Aetiology

Uncommon in nulliparous women, where it is due to congenital weakness of the pelvic supporting structures. The majority of women with prolapse have had children. Childbirth is associated with damage to the ligamentous tissues of the pelvis and nerve supply of the pelvic floor muscles, causing later weakness. Other factors contributing to or exacerbating these effects include postmenopausal atrophy of pelvic-supporting tissue and chronic raised intra-abdominal pressure, e.g. with obesity or chronic cough.

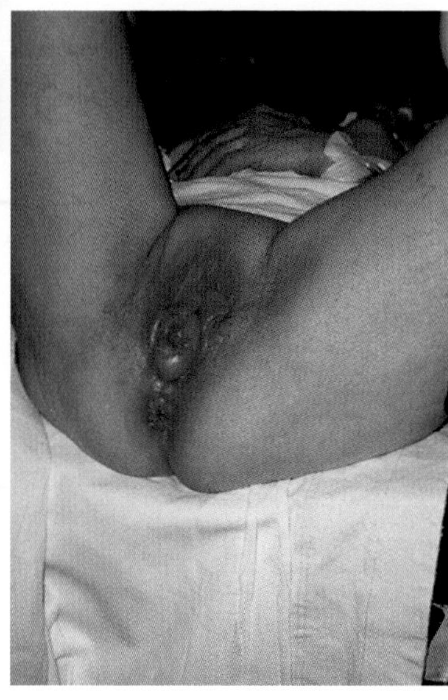
Fig. 139 Procidentia.

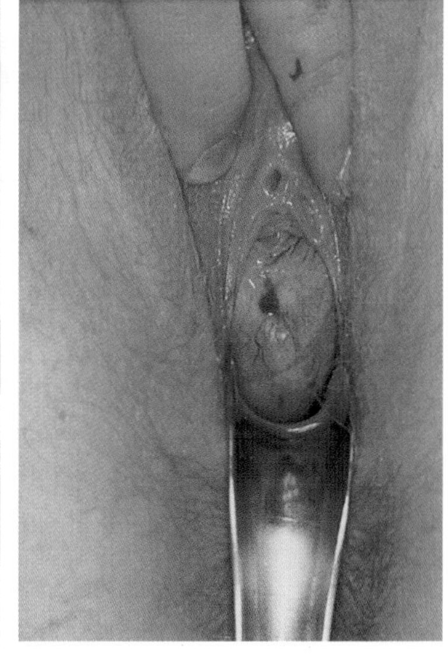
Fig. 140 Cystocele.

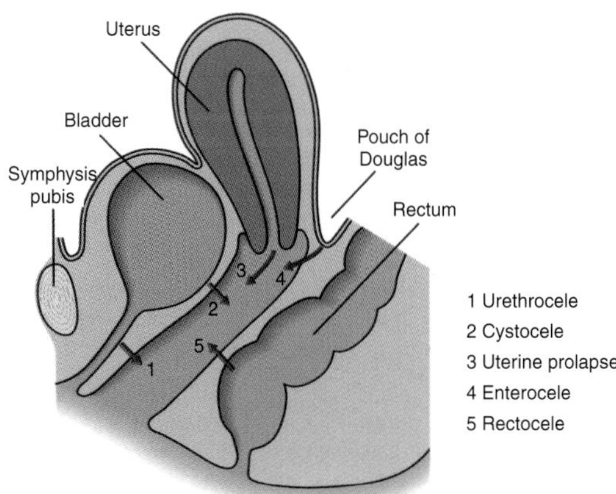

Fig. 141 Prolapse of the vagina.

Clinical features

Patients may describe a feeling of something 'coming down', and there is the presence of a lump protruding through the vulva. Urinary incontinence may be associated with a urethrocele. Urinary retention may be seen when a large cystocele is present. Difficulty with defaecation may also be present. Pain is not a feature of prolapse but dragging discomfort and backache that worsen throughout the day may be experienced.

Management

Prophylaxis Avoid traumatic vaginal deliveries and encourage antenatal and postnatal pelvic floor exercises. Discourage cigarette smoking and use hormone replacement therapy appropriately in postmenopausal women.

Conservative treatment Rings and shelf pessaries (Fig. 142) are a suitable short-term option in women unfit or not keen to undergo surgery, and between pregnancies.

Surgery Procedures include:

- *Anterior repair*: corrects a cystocele but may not be the most appropriate treatment for stress incontinence
- *Posterior repair*: corrects a rectocele
- *Vaginal hysterectomy*: is the treatment of choice in uterine prolapse and is combined with anterior and posterior repairs as necessary (Fig. 143).
- *Manchester (Fothergill) repair*: involves shortening the transverse cervical ligaments and amputating the cervix, together with an anterior repair. It is a useful operation when the uterine body is well supported, but the cervix is elongated and protruding

A vaginal vault prolapse occurring after hysterectomy can be corrected by a sacrospinous fixation or by securing the vagina to the sacrum abdominally or laparoscopically.

Complications

Long-term use of pessaries can cause vaginal ulceration. Immediate complications of vaginal surgery include haemorrhage, haematoma formation, infection and urinary retention. Wound breakdown and extrusion of bowel through the vagina (Fig. 144) are extremely rare. In the longer term, stenosis and dyspareunia may result. Prolapse may also recur.

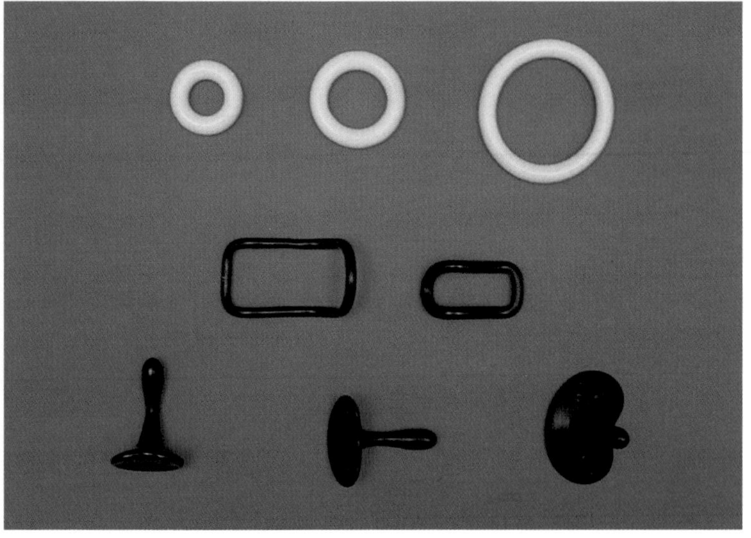

Fig. 142 Rings and shelf pessaries used to relieve prolapse.

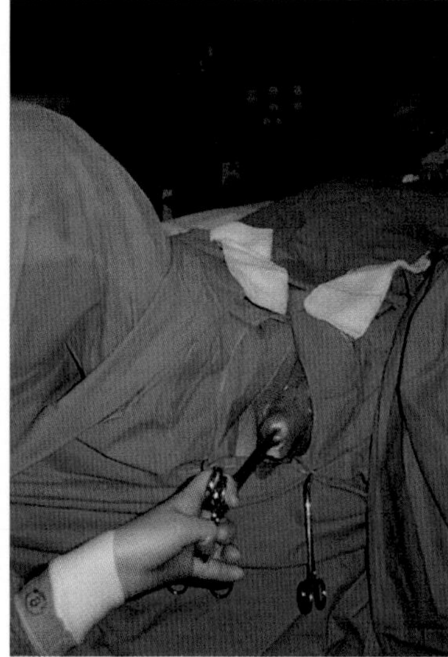

Fig. 143 Procidentia at commencement of vaginal hysterectomy.

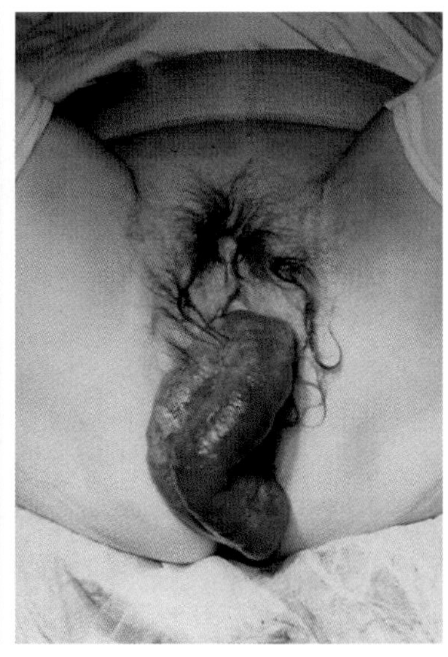

Fig. 144 Bowel herniation – a rare complication of vaginal hysterectomy.

19 Urinary incontinence

Urge incontinence

Definition

Involuntary loss of urine caused by uninhibited detrusor contractions.

Aetiology

Most cases are idiopathic. The detrusor contracts in an uninhibited fashion, causing urgency and frequency, and when the intravesical pressure exceeds the intraurethral pressure, incontinence results.

Clinical features

The history will reveal urinary frequency, urgency, nocturia and, perhaps, incontinence. On examination there is usually no abnormality.

Investigations

A mid-stream urine specimen should be taken for microscopy and culture. If there is any suggestion of a 'mixed' picture, i.e. symptoms of urge as well as stress, urodynamic investigations are essential (Fig. 145). Padweighing can be used to assess incontinence. Videocystourethrography is also useful (Fig. 146).

Management

Bladder drill This requires patient motivation and ideally biofeedback. The patient is told to pass urine at certain time intervals, which are then gradually increased until 3 or 4 h is reached.

Drug therapy Calcium antagonists, anticholinergic agents, ganglion blockers, oestrogen replacement and postganglion blockers.

Surgery Clam cystoplasty, bladder transection and sacral neurectomy are rarely used and are reserved for difficult cases.

Complications

Recurrence of symptoms is common. Bladder rupture can occur with cystodistension. Voiding difficulties can occur after surgery.

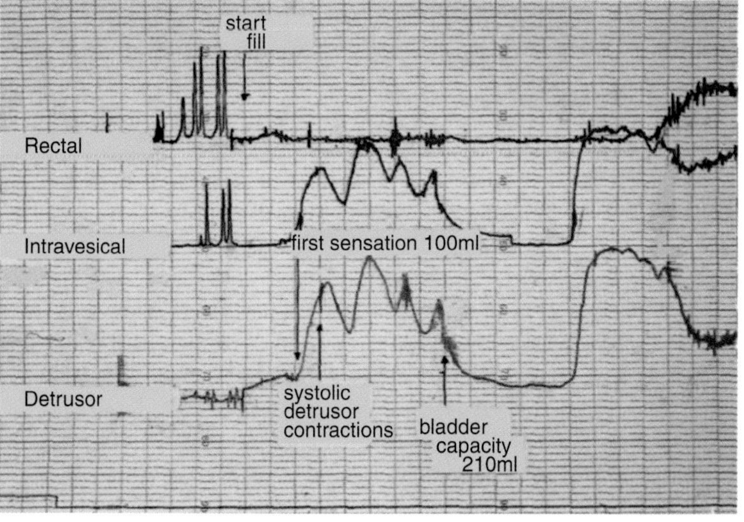

Fig. 145 Cystometry readout showing a stable bladder.

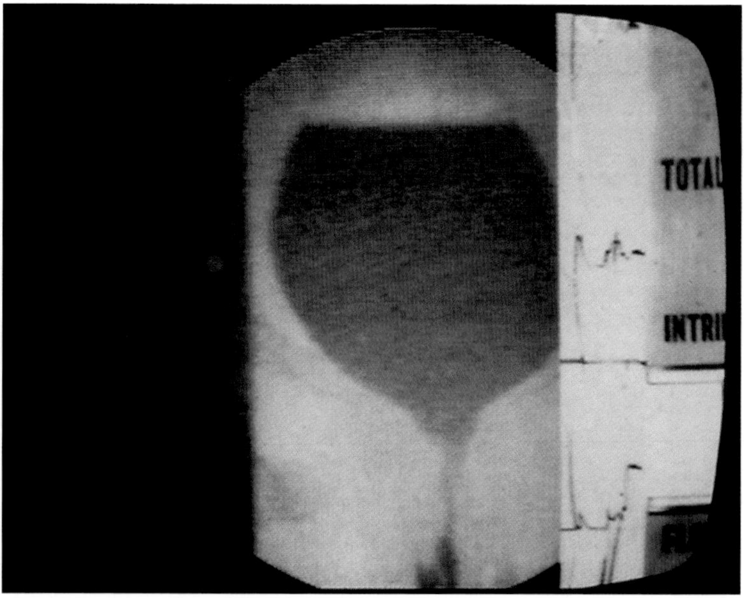

Fig. 146 Leakage of urine into bladder neck seen on videocystourethrography.

Genuine stress incontinence

Definition

Involuntary loss of urine when intra-abdominal pressure rises.

Aetiology

Urethral sphincter weakness, which is either congenital or secondary to multiparity, prolapse, menopause or previous surgery.

Clinical features

The patient gives a history of losing urine involuntarily when she laughs, coughs or sneezes. On examination the vulva may be excoriated due to persistent wetness. If the patient is placed in the Sims position and a Sims speculum is inserted to display the anterior vaginal wall, urine loss may be demonstrated when the patient is asked to cough (providing her bladder is not empty). A cystocele may be present.

Management

Infection should be treated. Other treatments include:

- *Physiotherapy:* involving pelvic floor exercises with cones (Fig. 147) or faradism can be effective
- *Colposuspension:* the bladder neck is elevated by inserting sutures beside the urethra and bladder neck. This can be done using an abdominal incision or laparoscopically.
- *Tension-free vaginal tape (TVT) procedure:* a knitted Prolene mesh tape is placed mid-urethra and is brought up through the anterior abdominal wall; the aim is to have the tape lying free at rest and only exerting sufficient pressure on the urethra during a cough to prevent leakage of urine (Fig. 148)
- *Anterior colporrhaphy:* the urethra is elevated from below after opening up the anterior vaginal wall
- *Injectables:* GAX collagen or macroplastique is injected paraurethrally to build up bulk around the sphincter
- *Slings:* organic or inorganic material is used.
- *Endoscopic bladder neck suspensions:* are useful for recurrent stress incontinence
- *Artificial sphincters*

Complications

Following surgery, voiding difficulties are common and recurrence of the stress incontinence is not uncommon. The results of surgery are poor if detrusor instability was present originally.

Prognosis

Colposuspensions have a 90% cure rate and anterior colporrhaphies 40–60%.

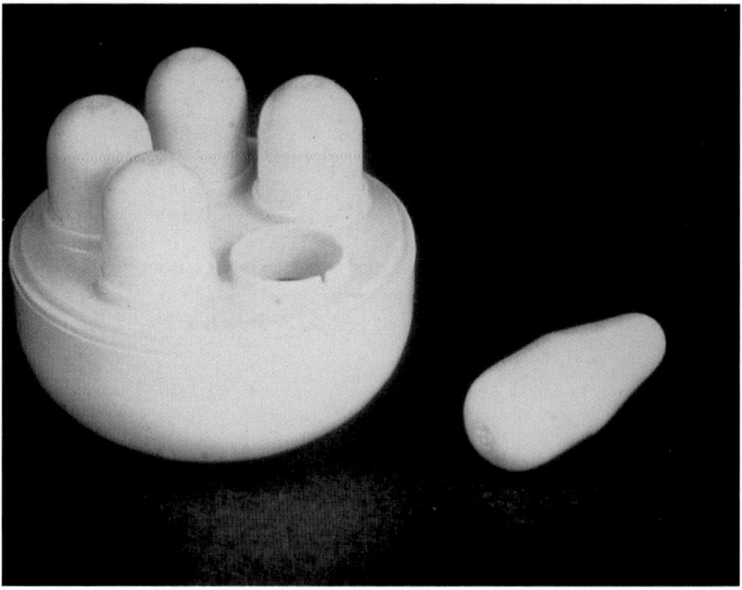

Fig. 147 Vaginal cones.

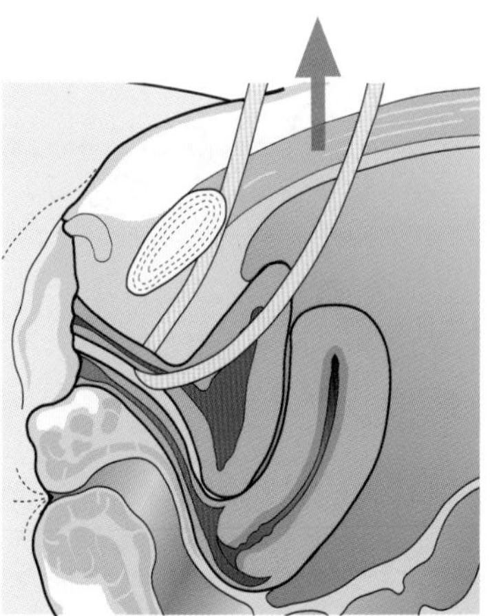

Fig. 148 Tension-free vaginal tape.

Overflow incontinence

Definition
Frequent involuntary loss of small volumes of urine, slow urinary stream and a postmicturition feeling of incomplete emptying.

Aetiology
Obstruction to bladder outflow in bladder atony which can be due to motor neurone lesions, drugs, surgery, pelvic mass, uterovaginal prolapse, local inflammation or immobilization.

Clinical features
History will reveal the above symptoms. Examination will demonstrate an enlarged bladder, and catheterization will produce a large residual volume of urine.

Investigations
MSU (mid-stream urine)

Cystometry will demonstrate a delayed first sensation and a large bladder capacity. Maximum voiding pressure will be normal or increased, and the peak flow rate will be slow. Micturating cystourethrogram (Fig. 149). Uroflowmeter.

Treatment
This will depend on the cause. Neurological causes are not treatable and intermittent self-catheterization can be learned.

True incontinence

Definition
Continuous incontinence.

Aetiology
Usually due to a fistulous track (Fig. 150) secondary to obstructed labour, surgery, carcinoma or radiotherapy.

Clinical features
There will be a history of continuous draining of urine from vagina. Examination may reveal the track, and colouring the urine may aid location.

Investigations
A micturating cystourethrogram and/or an IVP may help location.

Management
Conservative. Depending on aetiology, some may heal with time.

Surgery can be performed abdominally or vaginally. The fistulous track is removed and an interposition graft used if the tissues are poor.

Complications
Stress incontinence, vaginal scarring and recurrence.

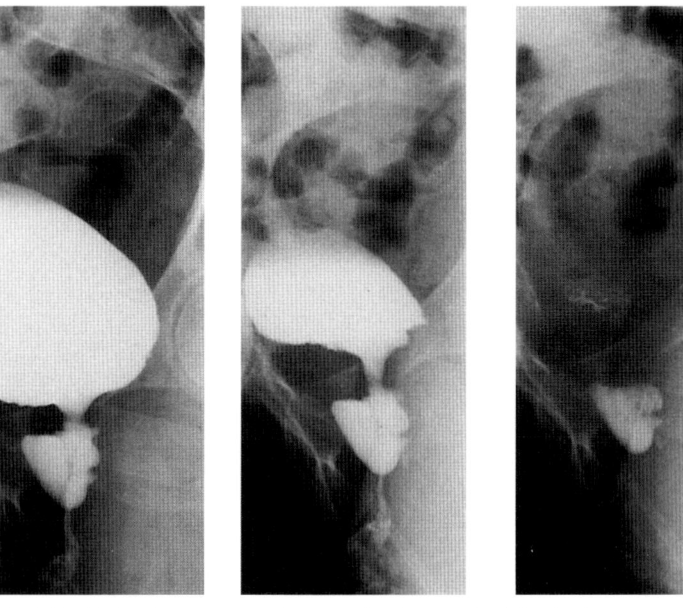

Fig. 149 Micturating cystogram demonstrating large urethral diverticulum.

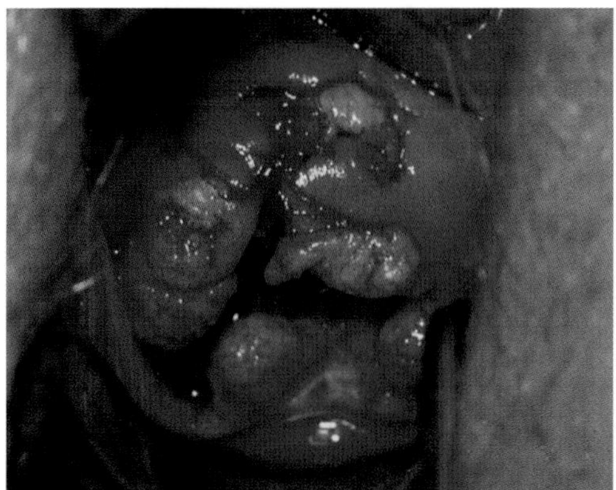

Fig. 150 Bladder mucosa visible through irregular fragments of vaginal mucosa.

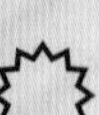

Questions

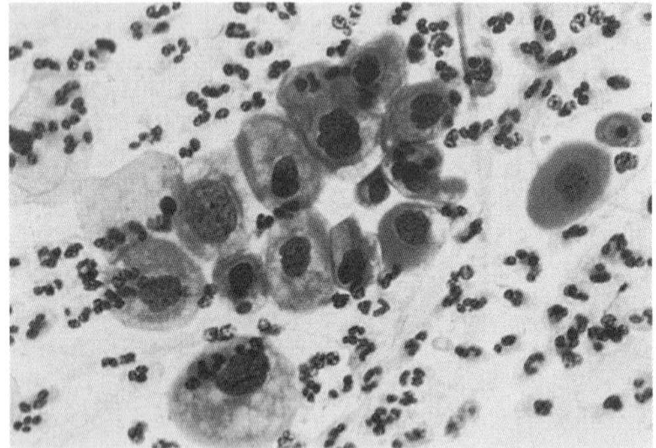

1. This slide shows dyskaryosis.

a. What type of cells are these?
b. These cells display some of the features of malignancy. Name them.
c. What is the management?

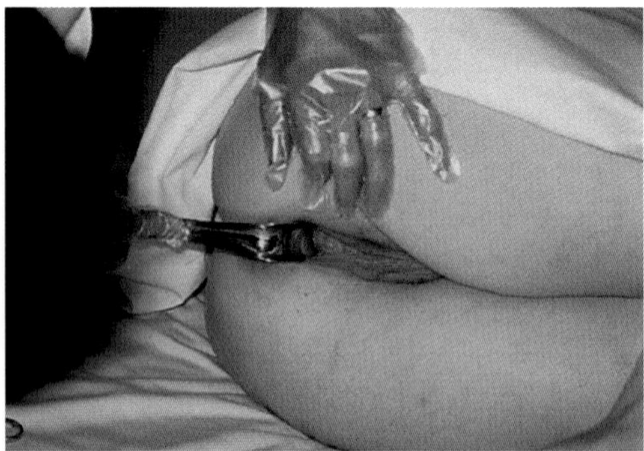

2.

a. What speculum is being used for this examination?
b. Describe the Sims position.
c. In what circumstances would you use this speculum?
d. What other instruments should you use with this speculum?

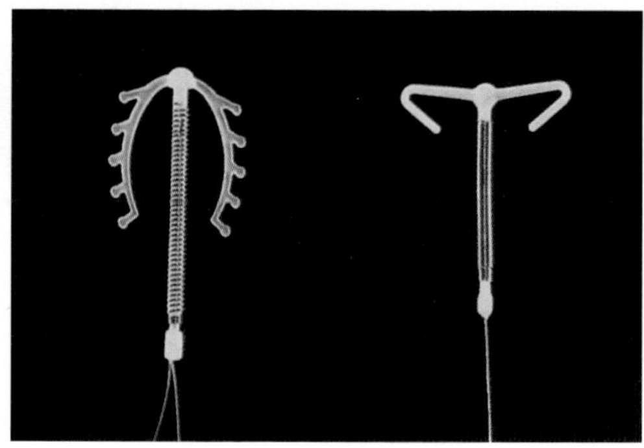

3.

a. What are these?
b. What is the mechanism of action?
c. What are the absolute contraindications?
d. Describe the mechanism of insertion.
e. What are the complications associated with their use?
f. How often should copper-containing devices be changed?

4.

a. What is the diagnosis?
b. What symptoms may the patient complain of?
c. How would you confirm the diagnosis?
d. What is the treatment?
e. How would you treat the recalcitrant case?

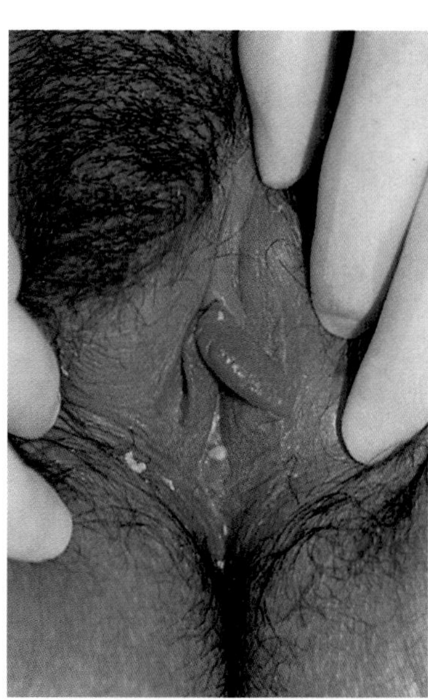

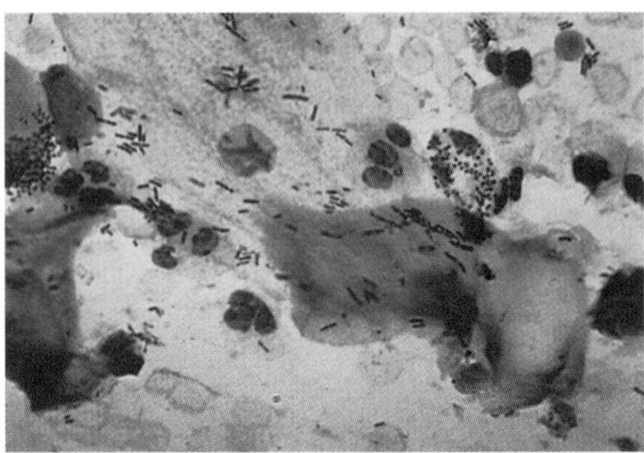

5.

a. What organisms are present on this Gram-stain smear?
b. What is the resultant clinical condition?
c. What are the clinical manifestations in females?
d. How is the definitive diagnosis made?
e. What are the principles of management?

6.

a. What procedure has this young girl undergone?
b. How may these patients present?
c. What problems can occur in labour?
d. What elective gynaecological procedure can alleviate the problem?
e. If diagnosed in labour how may delivery be facilitated?

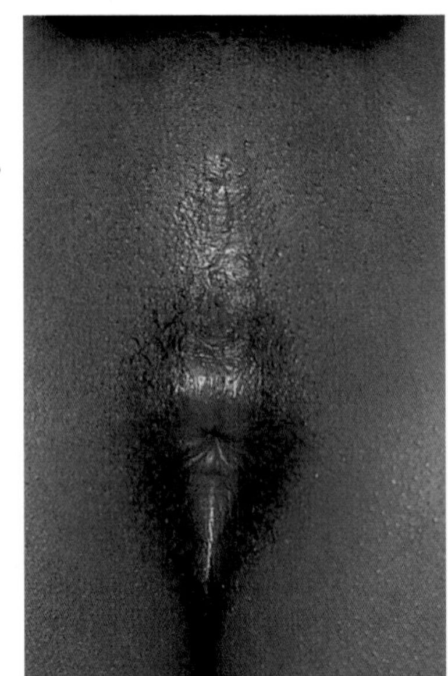

7.

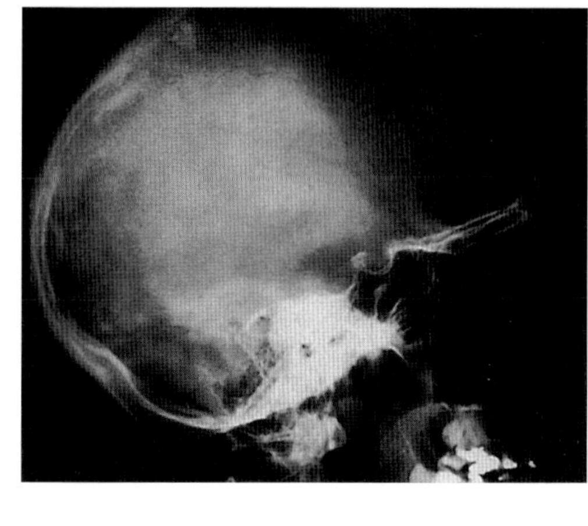

a. What does this X-ray reveal?
b. What other imaging techniques can be used to make the diagnosis?
c. What is the most likely cause and how would this patient present to the Gynaecology Department?
d. What other investigations would you perform?
e. Name other causes of hyperprolactinaemia.
f. What are the treatment options?

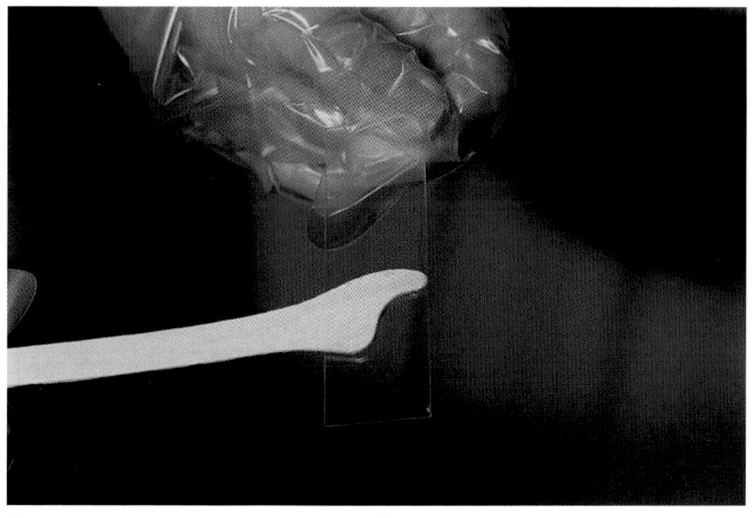

8.

a. What test is being performed and what is the purpose?
b. What is the name of the instrument?
c. How frequently should this investigation be performed?
d. What area must be sampled?
e. How can one optimize the sample obtained?

9.

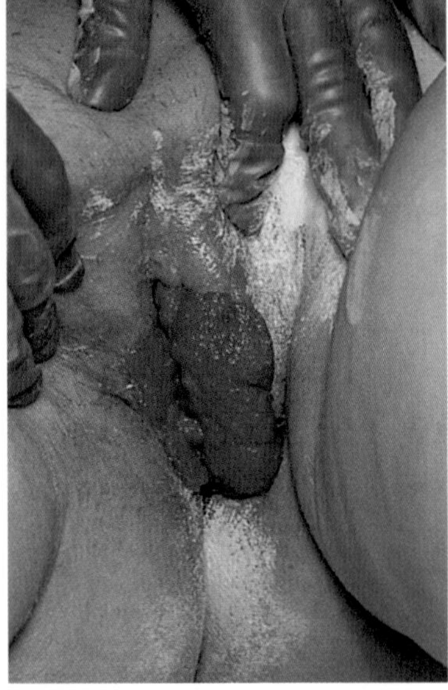

a. What is the obvious diagnosis?
b. In what age group does this condition typically occur?
c. What is the usual histology?
d. What is the primary route of spread?
e. What are the principles of treatment?

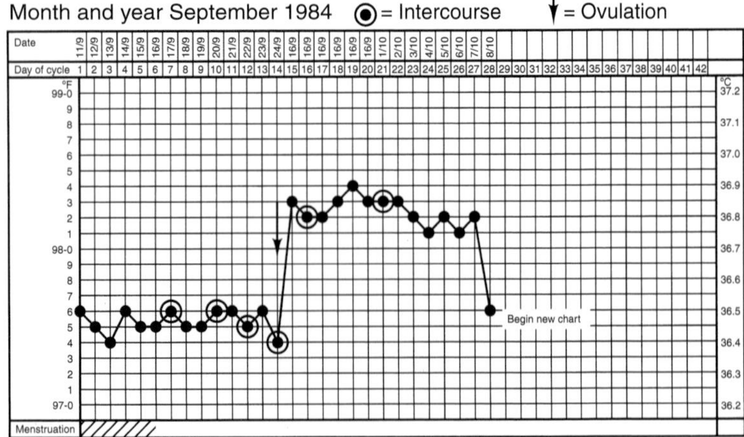

10.

a. What is the name of this record?
b. What does this record illustrate?
c. What event has presumptively occurred?
d. By what method can this event be more definitively diagnosed?

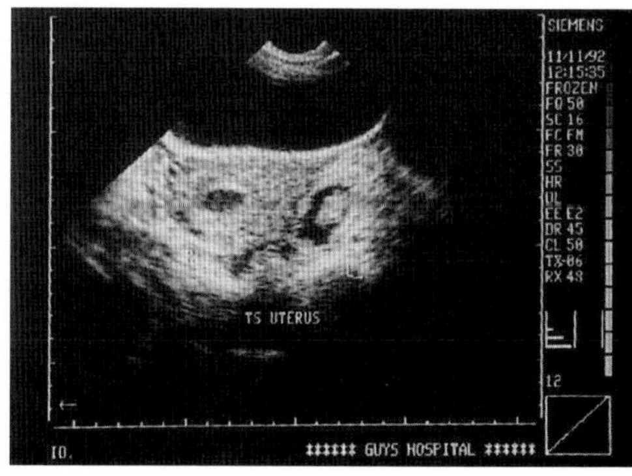

11. The photographs in questions 11–13 relate to a woman who presented with an unruptured ectopic pregnancy.

a. Describe the sonographic findings.
b. What are the classic symptoms of this condition?
c. What are the typical signs?
d. What ancillary investigations can help to make the diagnosis?

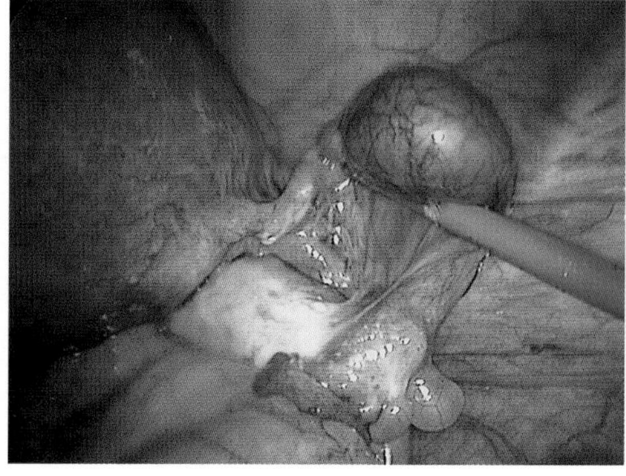

12.

a. What aetiological factors contribute to the incidence of ectopic pregnancy?
b. What are the common anatomical sites?
c. What is the natural history of ectopic pregnancy?
d. What is the differential diagnosis?

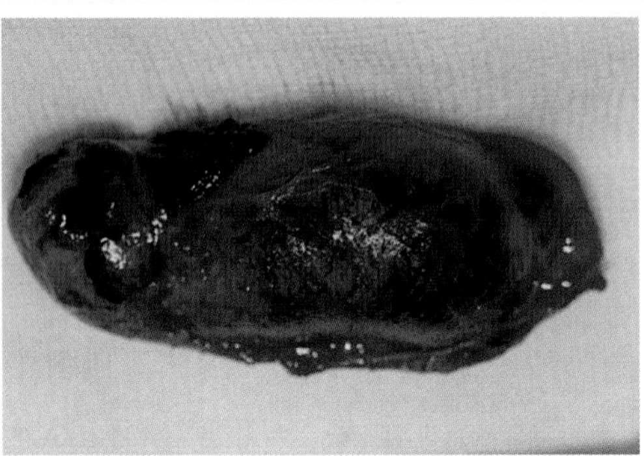

13. This patient underwent salpingectomy.

a. What treatment options are available in the treatment of ectopic pregnancies?
b. How would you counsel this patient postoperatively?
c. What is the recurrence risk?

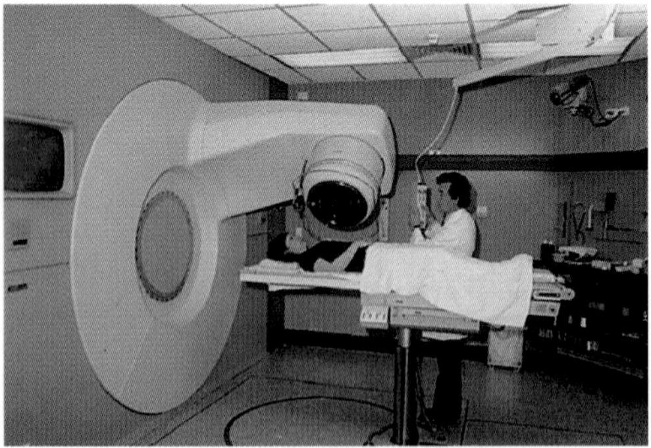

14. This young woman is undergoing radiation therapy.

a. For which gynaecological cancers does radiation therapy have an established curative role?
b. In what ways may radiation therapy be delivered?
c. What acute adverse reactions are seen?
d. What are the possible long-term sequelae of radiation therapy to the pelvic region?

15.

a. What is the most likely diagnosis? Define this condition.
b. What are the theories of aetiology?
c. What are the symptoms and signs?
d. How could the diagnosis be confirmed in this case?

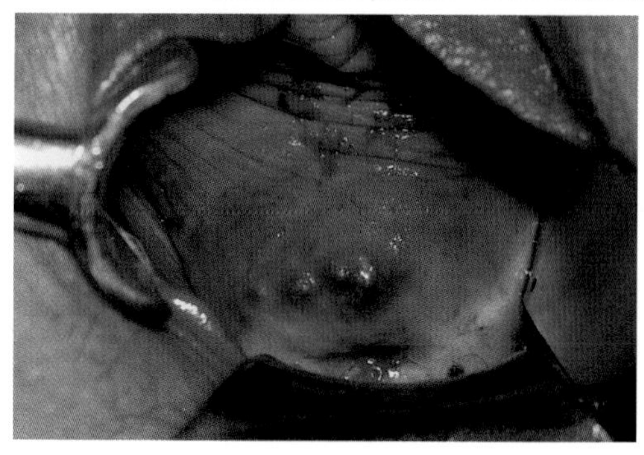

16.

a. Describe what you see.
b. What is the diagnosis?
c. What is the basis of this condition?
d. When do these patients normally present?
e. What else might you find on clinical examination?

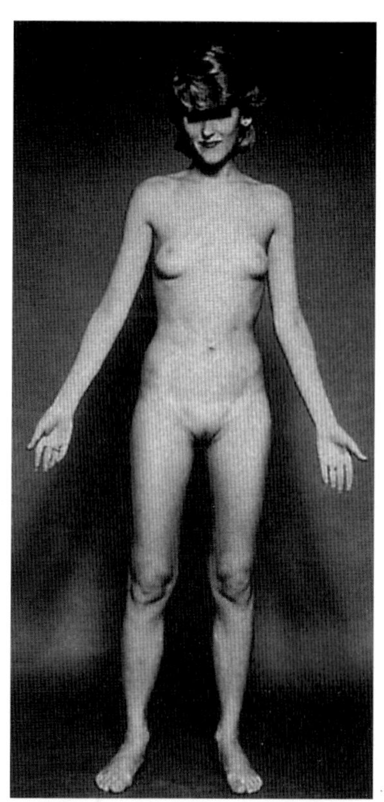

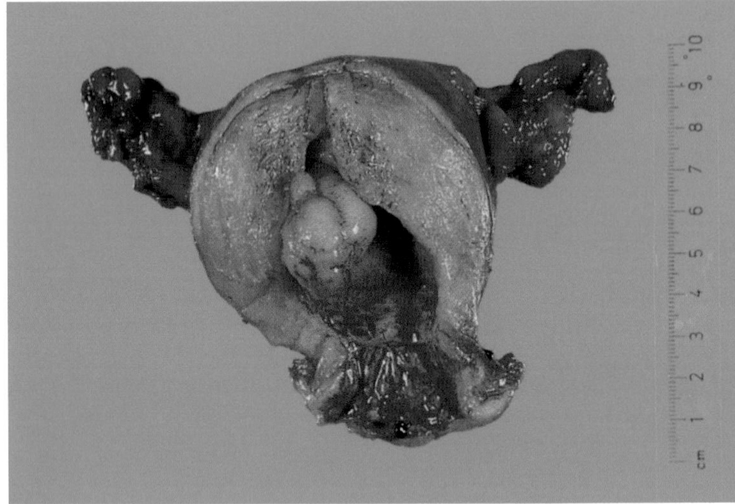

17.

a. Describe what you see.
b. What symptoms may these cause?
c. How may these be detected?
d. What is the treatment?

18. This woman is receiving depot medroxy progesterone acetate.

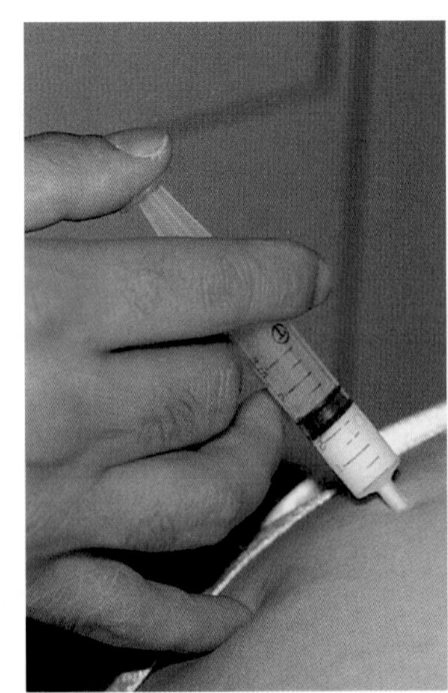

a. How does it work?
b. Is a steady dose provided?
c. What is the failure rate of this method?
d. What are the advantages of this method?
e. What are the disadvantages?

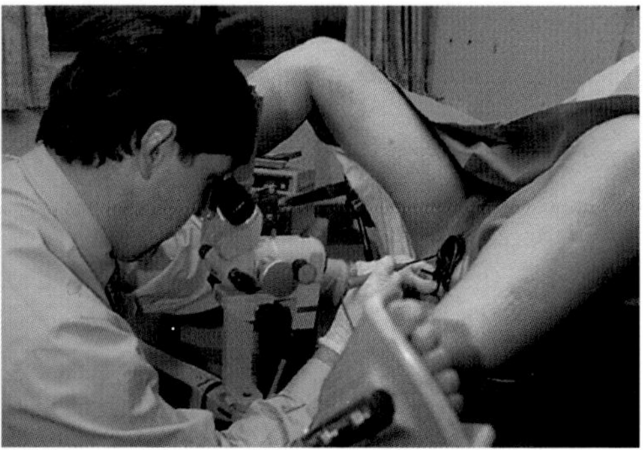

19.

a. What investigation is this woman undergoing?
b. Who would you refer for this investigation?
c. What basic steps are involved in this procedure?
d. How would you counsel a woman prior to referral?

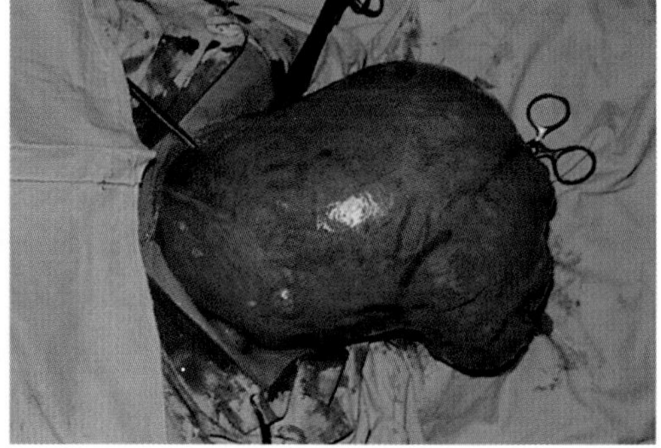

20. **This is an intraoperative specimen of a woman who had iron-deficiency anaemia.**

a. What might have caused this anaemia?
b. What symptoms might she have presented with?
c. What preoperative medication can be prescribed to simplify surgery?

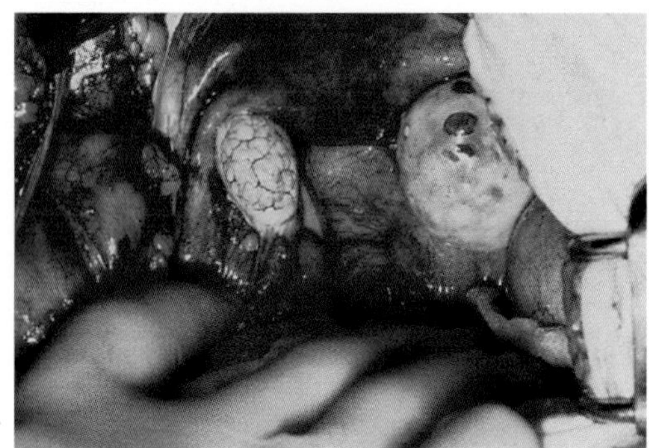

21.

a. Outline the diagnostic approach in a patient who exhibits virilism.
b. What cause of virilism is present in this patient?
c. Which ovarian tumours produce androgens and virilizing syndromes?
d. Which signs of virilism disappear after removal of such tumours?

22.

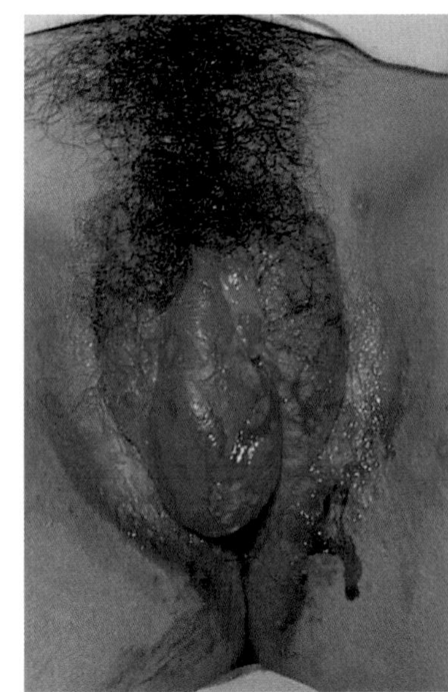

a. What is the diagnosis?
b. What are the typical clinical features?
c. How should this condition be managed?
d. What are the obstetric implications of this condition?

23.

a. What is the diagnosis?
b. What is the age distribution of this condition?
c. What is the typical presentation?
d. What is the characteristic pattern of spread?
e. How is this condition staged?
f. Define the four stages.

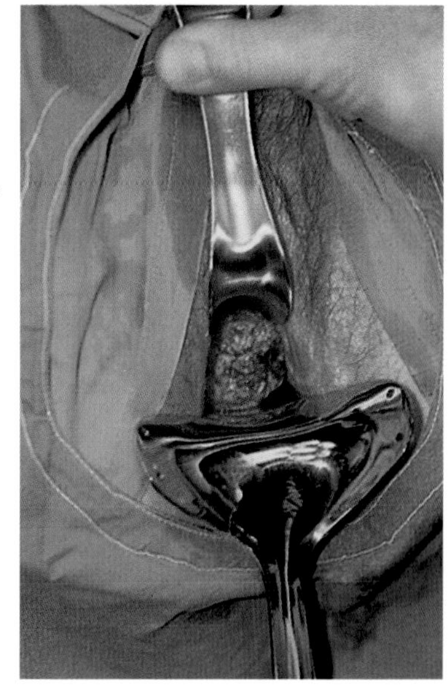

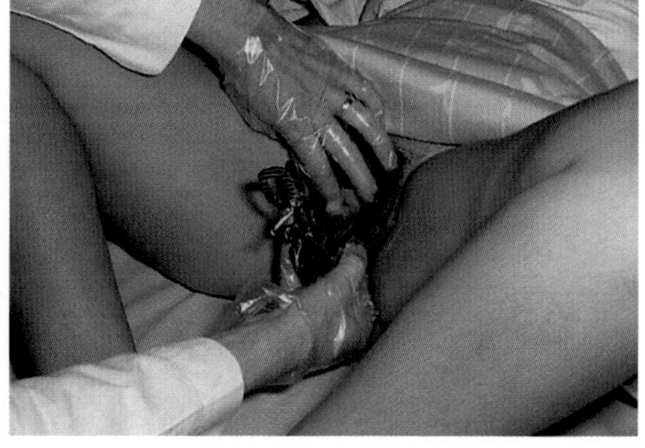

24.

a. What is this speculum called?
b. What position is the patient in?
c. How would you insert this speculum?
d. What examination would you use as an adjunct to the use of this speculum?

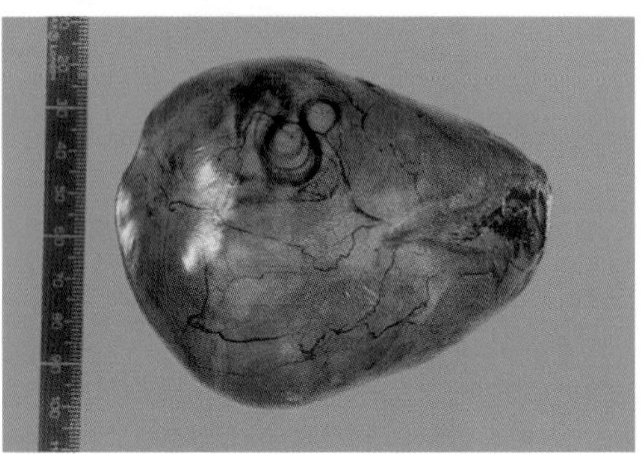

25.

a. What is the diagnosis?
b. At what ages is this typically seen?
c. What is the origin of the cyst? What tissues can be within it?
d. What is the incidence of bilateral lesions and what is the significance of this figure?
e. What is the malignant potential?

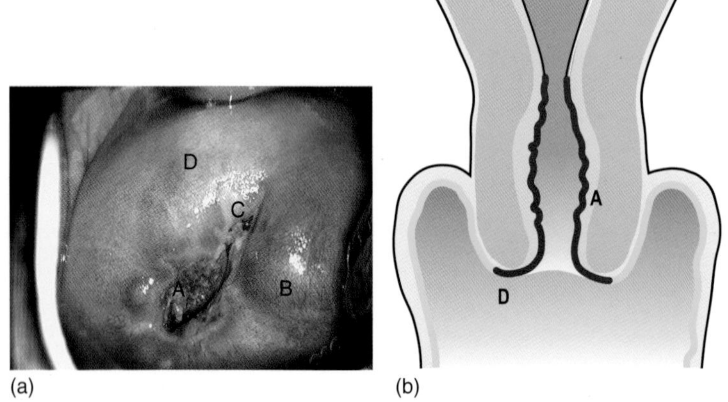

(a) (b)

26. Identify the four areas labelled on the cervix.

27.

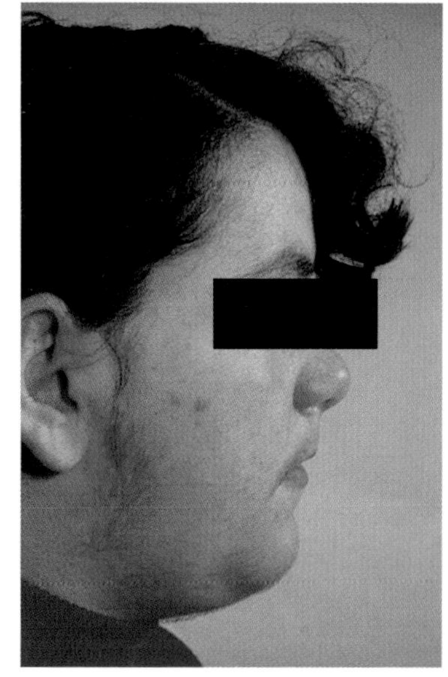

a. What is the name of this condition?
b. What scoring system can help estimate the severity of the problem?
c. What are the common causes?
d. How would you investigate this patient?
e. What treatment modalities are available?

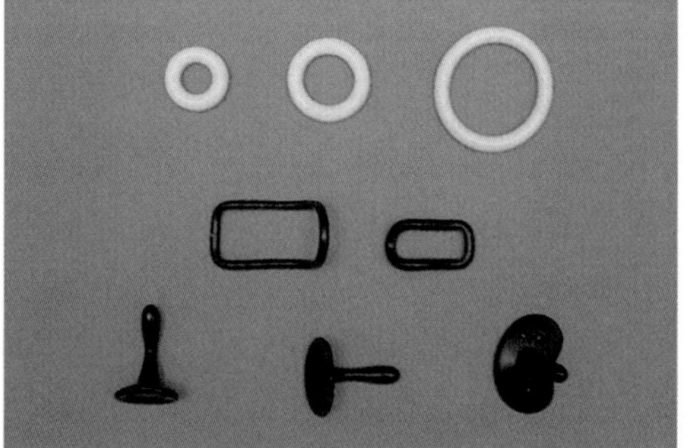

28.

a. What are these devices called?
b. Name the three types illustrated.
c. What are the indications for their use?
d. What potential complications can occur with their use?
e. How often should the white devices be changed?

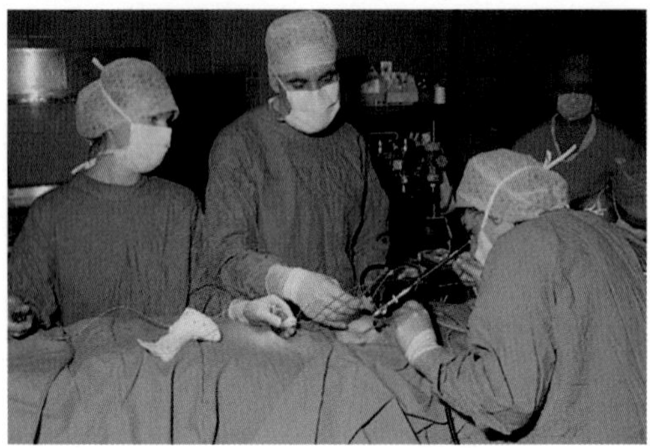

29.

a. What procedure is being performed?
b. What is the peritoneal cavity inflated with?
c. What organs can be visualized by this method?
d. What must be done before the Veress needle is introduced?

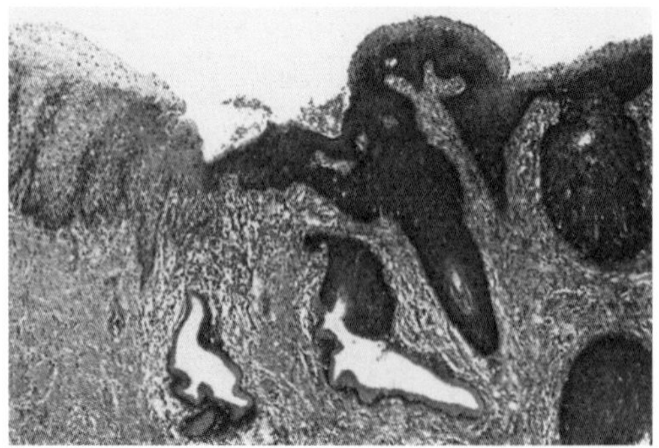

30. This is a slide of a cervix.

a. What does it show?
b. Is there evidence of invasion?
c. If the lesion was completely excised by cone biopsy, what follow-up would you arrange?
d. Prior to treatment what would you anticipate the smear on this woman to reveal?

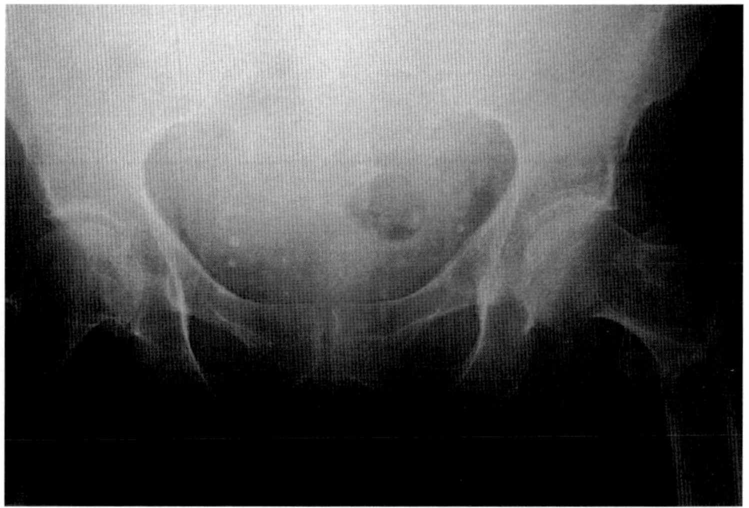

31.

a. What does this photograph show?
b. Name the probable underlying pathology.
c. What other sites are affected by the underlying pathology?
d. What are the causes of the underlying problem?
e. What are the long-term implications for this woman's health?

32.

a. What are the two diagnoses present?
b. What are the usual symptoms?
c. What are the risk factors for the underlying disease?
d. What type of bone predominates in the spine?
e. What are the lifestyle implications for the conditions illustrated?

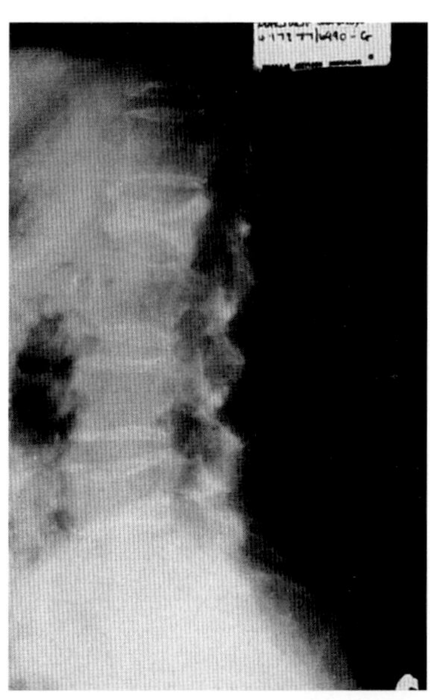

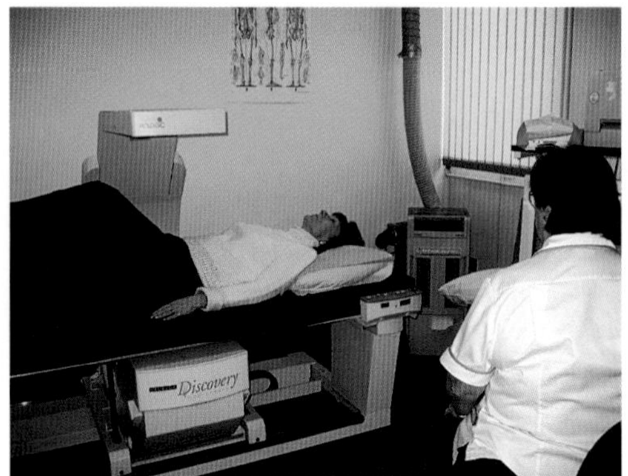

33.

a. What is this examination?
b. At what age does a woman attain peak bone mass?
c. What measures can help to maximize the peak bone mass?
d. What is the age-related rate of bone loss?
e. What is the rate of bone loss following the menopause?

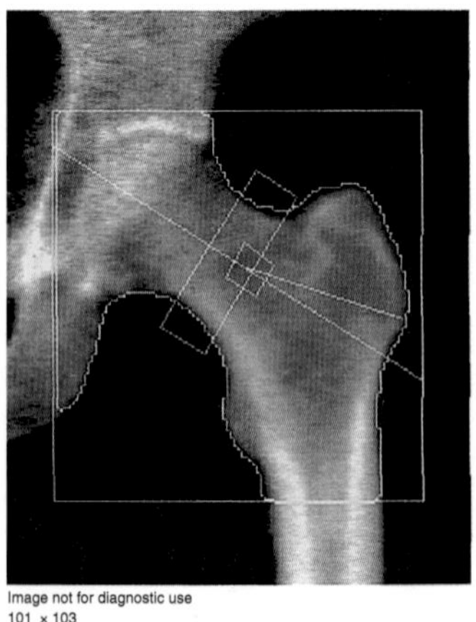

Scan Information:
Scan Date: 21 April 2004 ID: F0421040K
Scan Type: a Left Hip
Analysis: 21 April 2004 10:16 Version 12.1
Left Hip
Operator: PRM

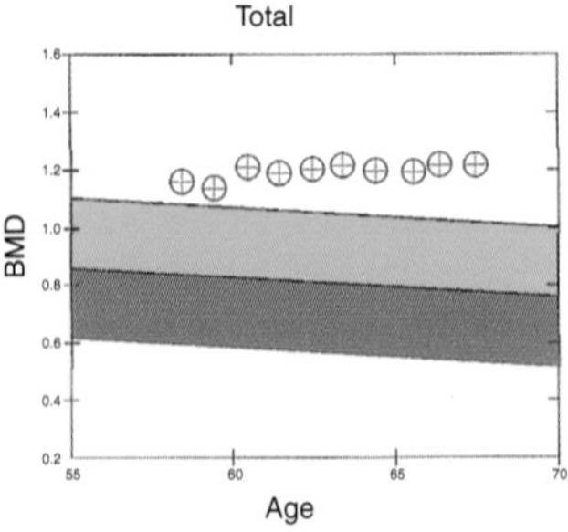

34.

a. How was this image produced?
b. What is being measured?
c. What other tests are available to obtain this measurement?
d. What is Ward's triangle?
e. What are the advantages of this test over the other methods?

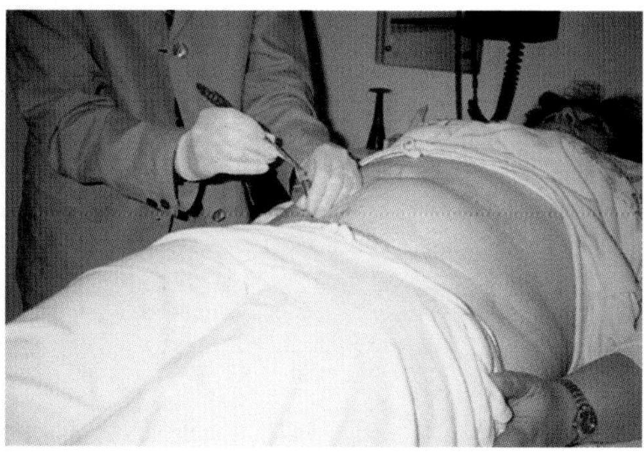

35.

a. What is the procedure that is being performed?
b. What is the likely ingredient?
c. Why are these administered?
d. How often are they administered?
e. Should progestogens be given as well?

36.

a. What is this condition?
b. What is the characteristic karyotype?
c. What are the typical physical findings?
d. Is spontaneous pregnancy a possibility for this person?
e. How can this condition be diagnosed antenatally?

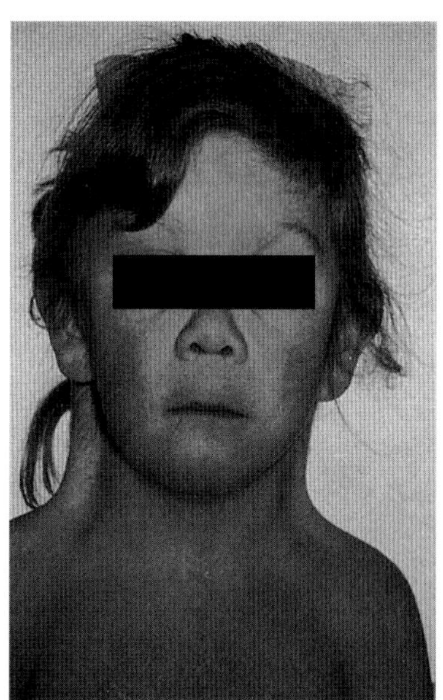

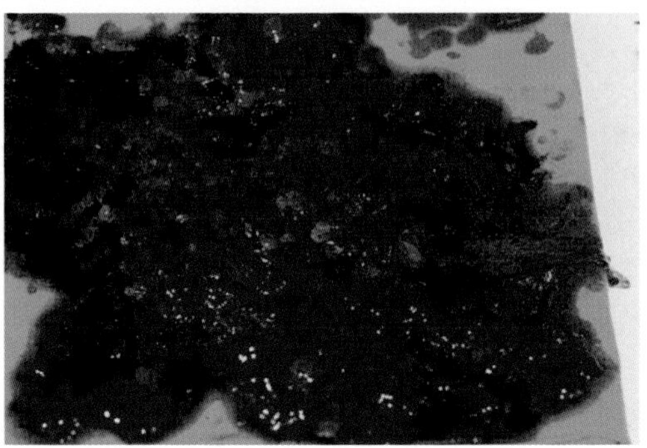

37. This tissue was removed at a D&C.

a. What does this illustrate?
b. What is the diagnosis?
c. What are the typical symptoms?
d. What are the signs?
e. What is the management?

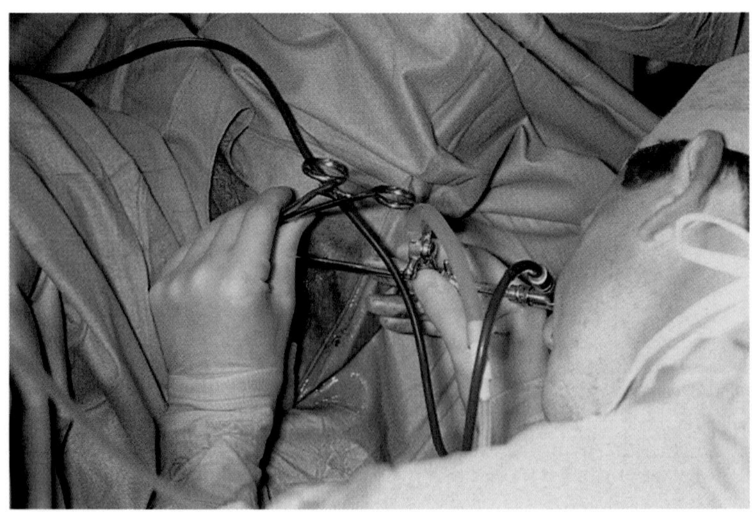

38. This woman presented with postmenopausal bleeding.

a. What investigation is being performed?
b. What is being passed through the rubber tubing?
c. What does this operation enable you to do?

39.

a. What investigation has been performed?
b. Describe the findings.
c. With what urinary symptoms may this patient present?
d. What gynaecological causes may result in this picture?

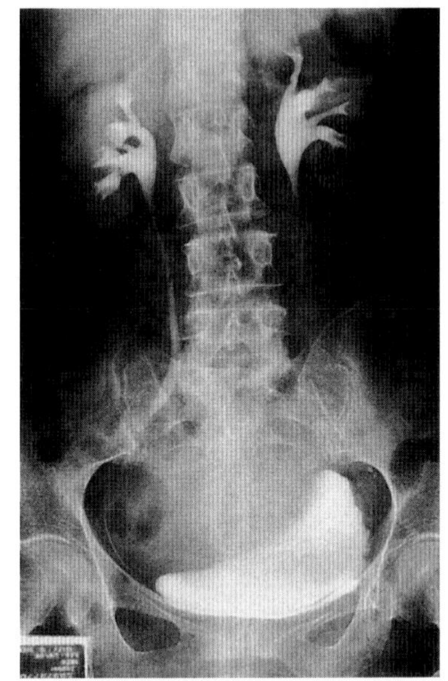

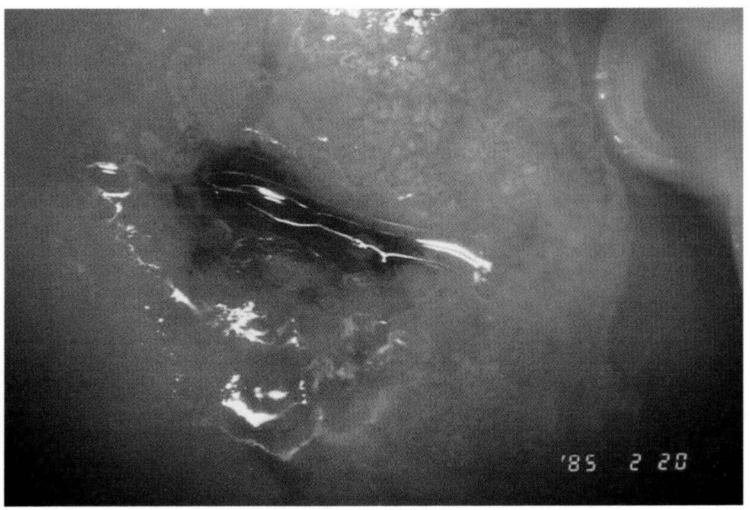

40.

a. What solution has been used on the cervix?
b. What can you see?
c. Do you think this is a severe or a minor lesion?
d. A biopsy showed CIN I. Describe CIN I.
e. Can spontaneous regression occur?

Semen analysis report

Normal values for our laboratory are given in brackets: they are based on specimens received within 1 hour of ejaculation and produced after 3 to 5 days of abstinence.

Clinical data: Subfertility Investigation

Patient DOB: 24/12/69

Time produced: 10:10 hr | **Time at lab:** 10:15hr

Abstinence: 6 days | **Volume:** 2.5ml (normal 2–5 ml)

pH: 7.5 (normal 7.2–7.8)

Sperm count: 67 million/ml (normal 20–300 million/ml)

Sperm motility (more than 50% should be motile after 1 hr)
75% at start
70% after 1 hr

Sperm morphology (less than 50% abnormal forms should be present)
58% normal forms
42% abnormal forms

41.

a. Is this result normal or abnormal?
b. What instructions would you give for collection?
c. What is a postcoital test?
d. Explain a positive and negative postcoital test.

42. This patient presented with secondary amenorrhoea.

a. Define secondary amenorrhoea.
b. Divide the causes of amenorrhoea into anatomical compartments.
c. What is the likely cause in this patient? What compartment is affected?
d. What baseline investigations would you perform?

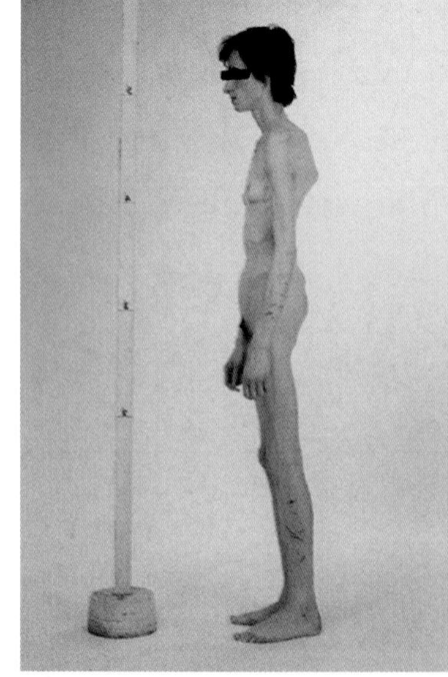

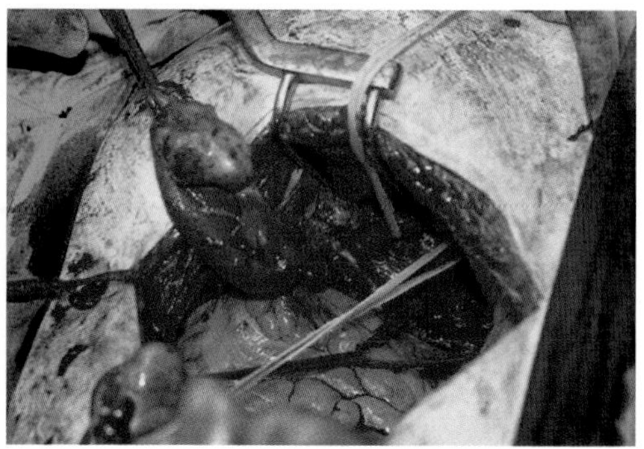

43. **The illustrations in questions 43 and 44 relate to Wertheim's hysterectomy.**

a. What two options are available for the first line treatment of cervical carcinoma?
b. What factors determine the choice of treatment?
c. What structures are removed?
d. What structures have been isolated by the uppermost and lowermost tapes?

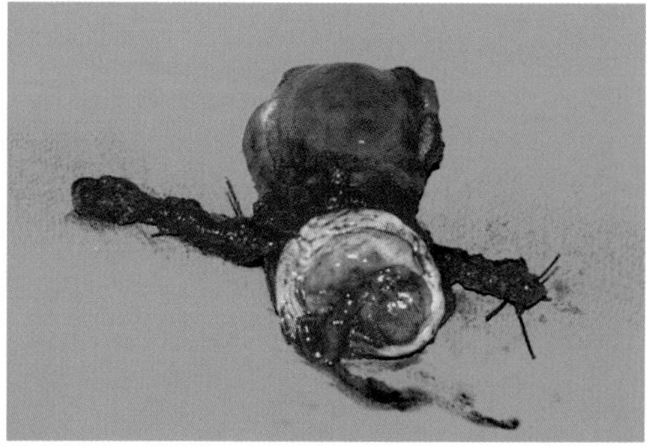

44.

a. What are the indications for a Wertheim's hysterectomy?
b. What lymph node groups are dissected during the procedure?
c. What are the complications of a Wertheim's hysterectomy?
d. What are the relative merits of the surgical approach and radiation therapy?

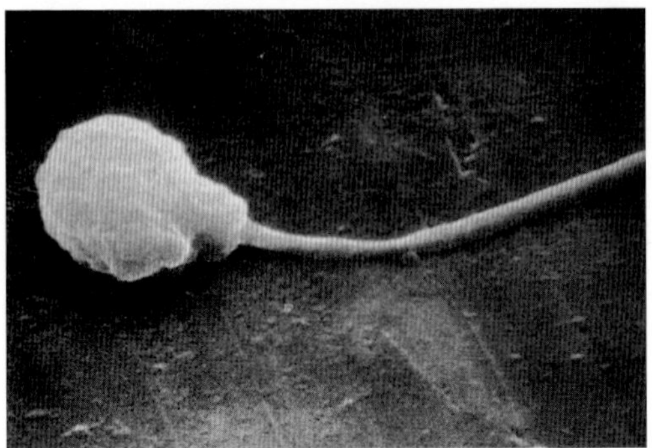

45.

a. What does this electron scanning micrograph illustrate?
b. What are the structural components?
c. Where is this structure produced?
d. What is the stimulus for its production?
e. What is the function of the Leydig cells?

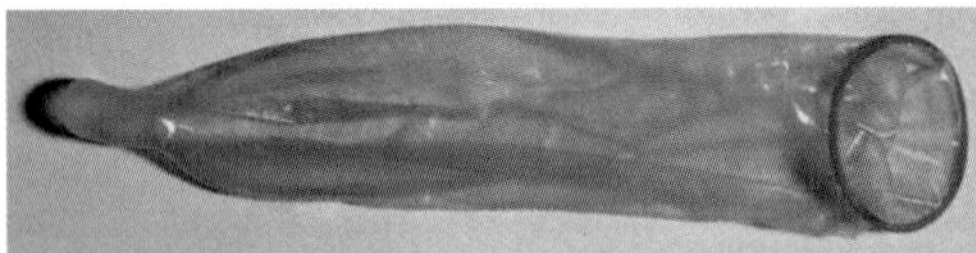

46.

a. What is the failure rate of condoms?
b. Describe the method of application and removal.
c. What are the advantages of this device?
d. If this device 'bursts', what is the management?

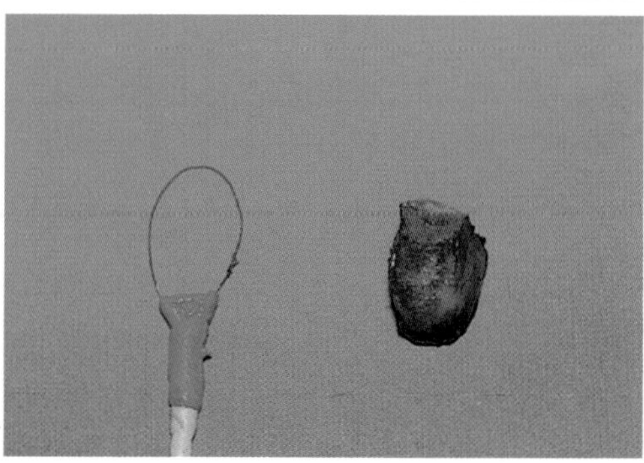

47.

a. What is the name of this specimen and instrument?
b. What is the purpose of this procedure?
c. What investigations should precede this procedure?
d. What alternative procedures are available?
e. What complications can follow this procedure and what advice would you give to the patient?

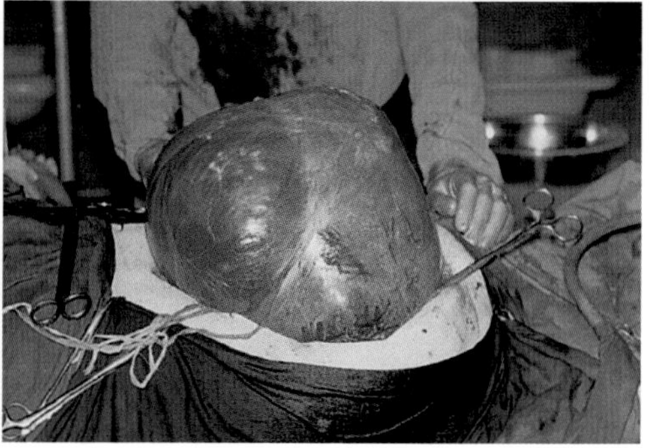

48. This abdominal mass was removed from an elderly woman.

a. With what symptoms may this woman have presented?
b. On examination, what signs would help with the differential diagnosis?
c. What investigations would you order?
d. How is the definitive diagnosis made?
e. What is the most likely gynaecological diagnosis?

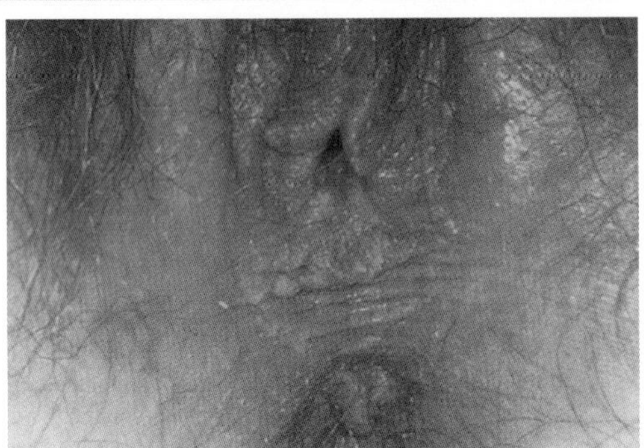

49.

a. What term describes this appearance?
b. What is the aetiological agent?
c. How is this condition usually acquired?
d. What modes of therapy are available?
e. How would you counsel this patient following treatment?

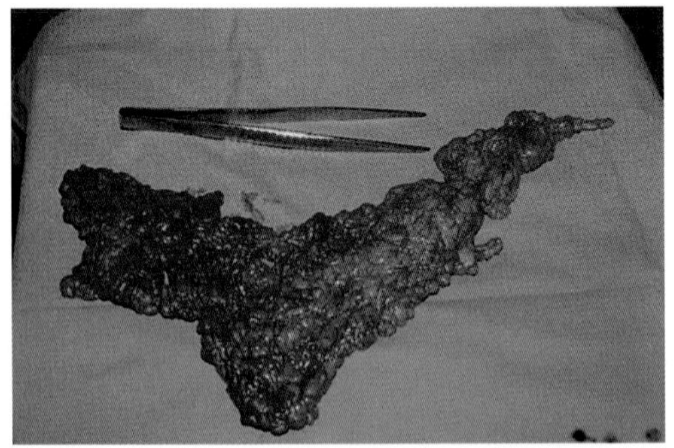

50. This specimen was removed at omentectomy.

a. What was the likely primary medical condition?
b. What is the typical pattern of spread of the primary condition?
c. Why was the above specimen removed?
d. What factors influence the prognosis of the primary condition?

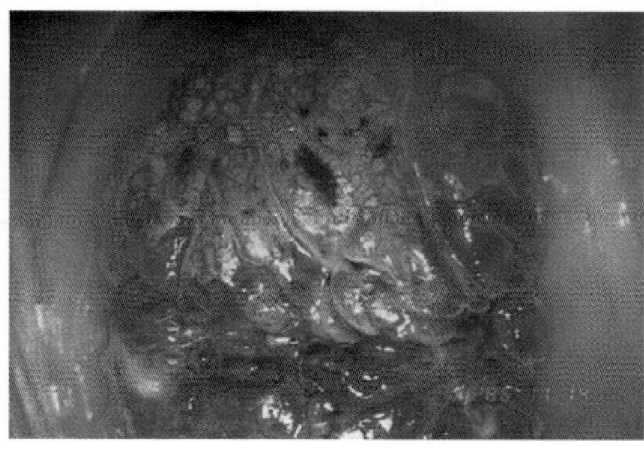

51. This cervix has been stained with acetic acid.

a. Describe what you see.
b. What does this colposcopic appearance suggest?
c. What would be your management?
d. Can these changes spontaneously revert to normal?

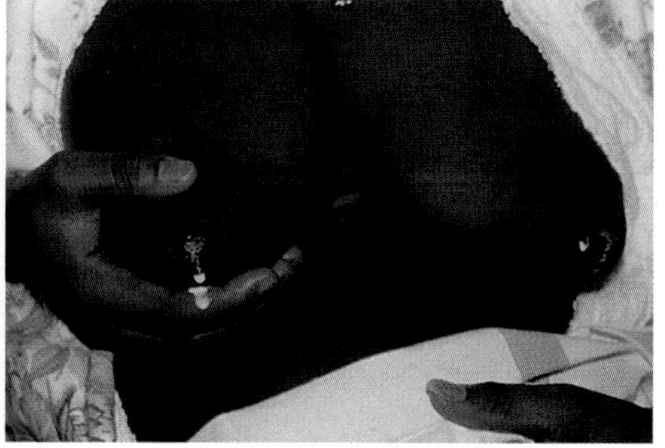

52.

a. Describe what you see.
b. What is this condition called?
c. What gynaecological condition may she have presented with?
d. What investigations would you perform?

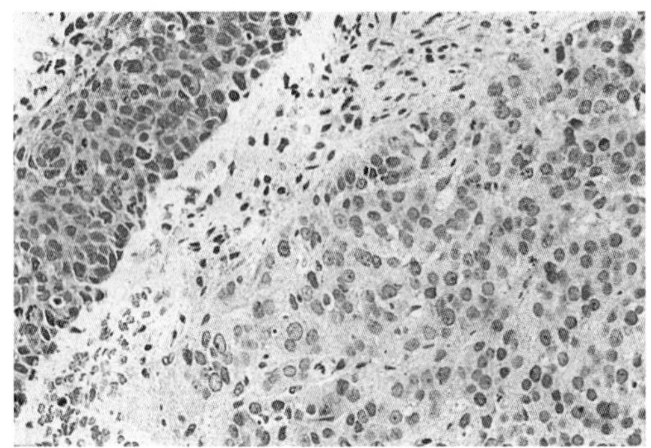

53. **This histology slide shows a section of cervix.**

a. What can you see?
b. What operation should be performed?
c. Could this woman have HRT when she is postmenopausal?

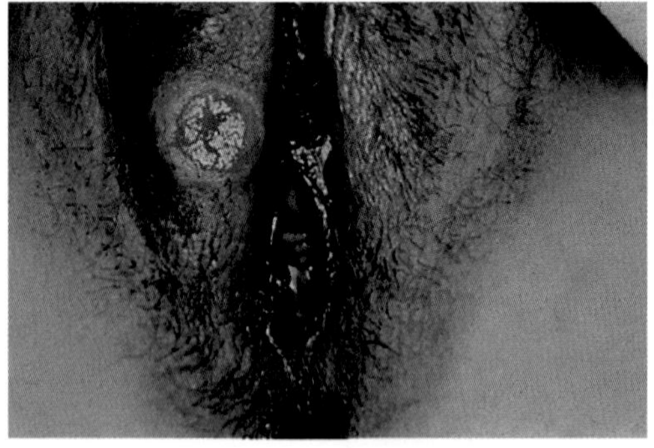

54.

a. What is the diagnosis?
b. Name the causative organism.
c. At what time does the illustrated lesion develop?
d. How is the definitive diagnosis made?
e. How should the illustrated condition be managed?

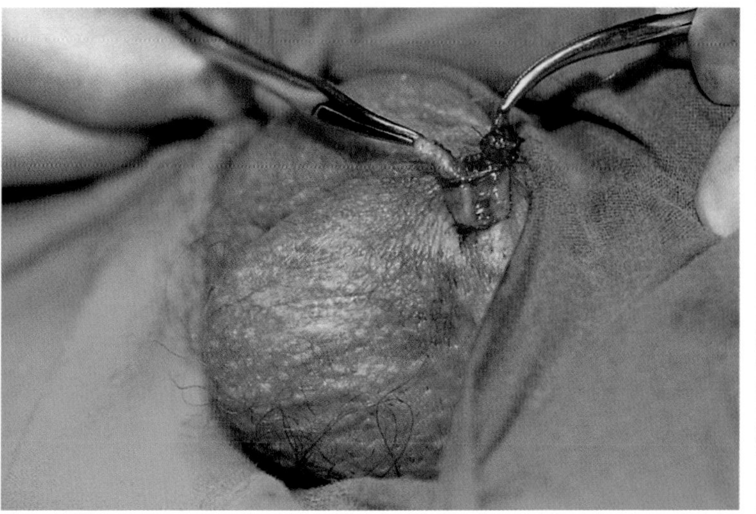

55.

a. What structure has been isolated?
b. What is the name of this operation?
c. What issues should be discussed in the preoperative counselling?
d. What are the complications of this operation?

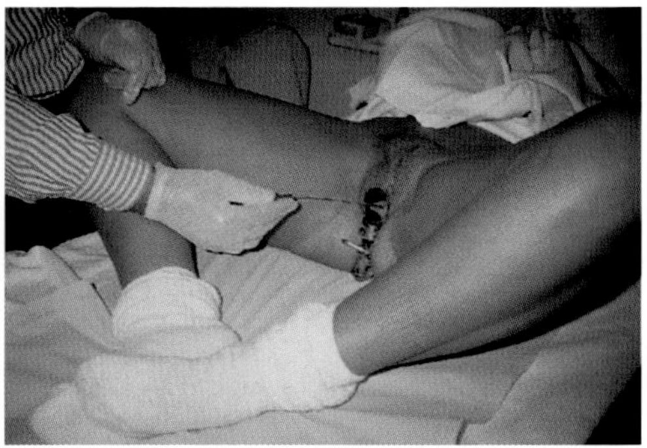

56.

a. What is the nature and purpose of this procedure?
b. What analgesia is required?
c. What are the contraindications?
d. How is this procedure performed?
e. What are the possible adverse reactions?

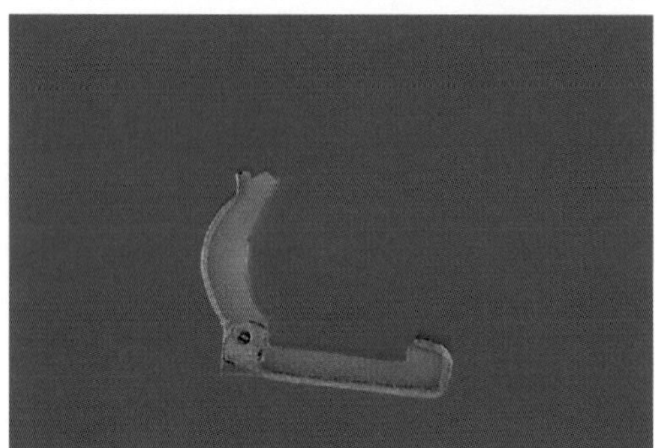

57.

a. What is this?
b. What is it used for?
c. How would you counsel the patient prior to the procedure?
d. What is the failure rate?

58.

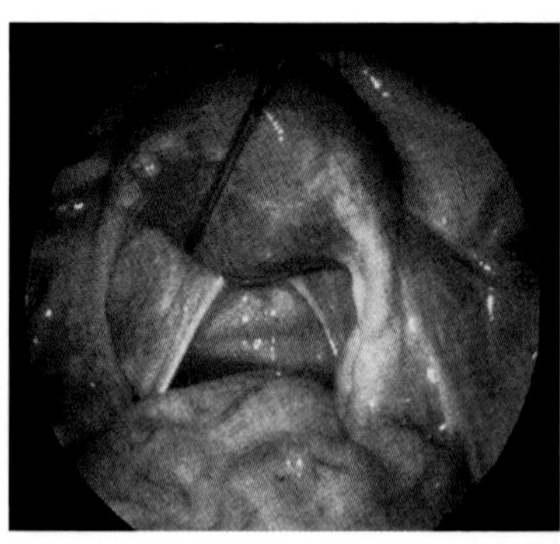

a. What structure is the probe supporting?
b. What are the white band-like structures in the centre portion of the photograph?
c. Is the free fluid that is seen necessarily pathological?
d. What structure occupies the posterior one-third of the illustration?

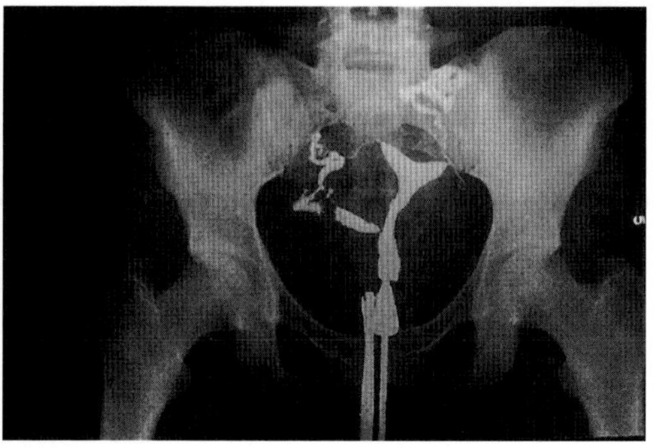

59.

a. What is the investigation?
b. What are the indications for this investigation?
c. What are the risks of this procedure?
d. What does this investigation show?

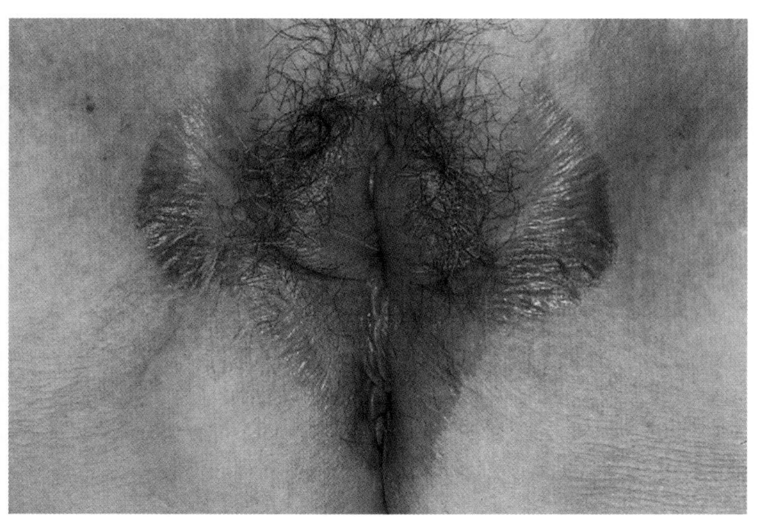

60. This woman presented with pruritus vulvae.

a. What are the possible causes?
b. How is the diagnosis made?
c. Describe a typical regime for treatment of the above.

61.

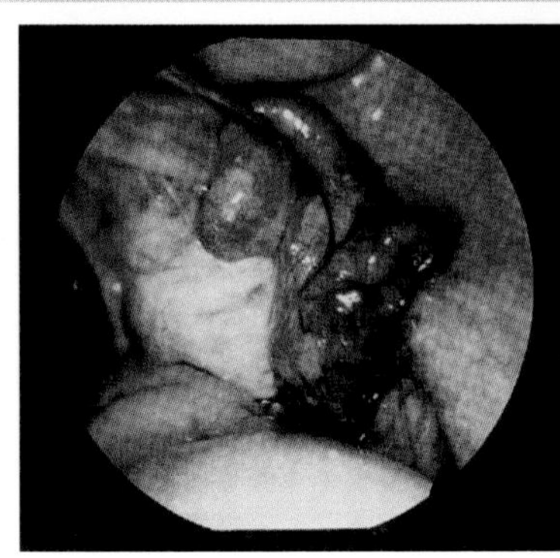

a. What operation has been performed?
b. What are the main indications for this procedure?
c. What are the relative merits for this procedure in comparison to hysterosalpingography?
d. What comment would you make concerning this patient's tubes?

62.

a.–e. Name the five types of miscarriage.

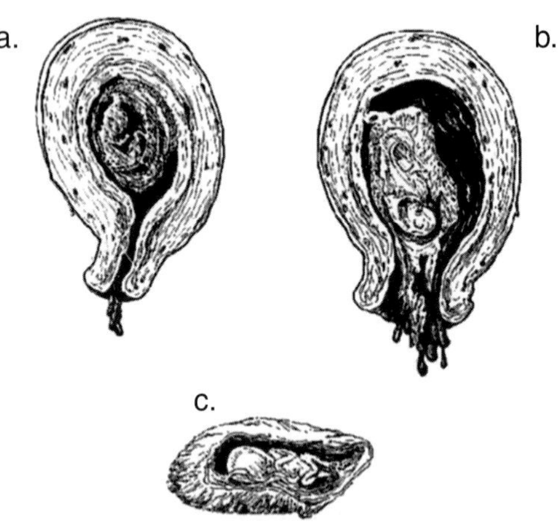

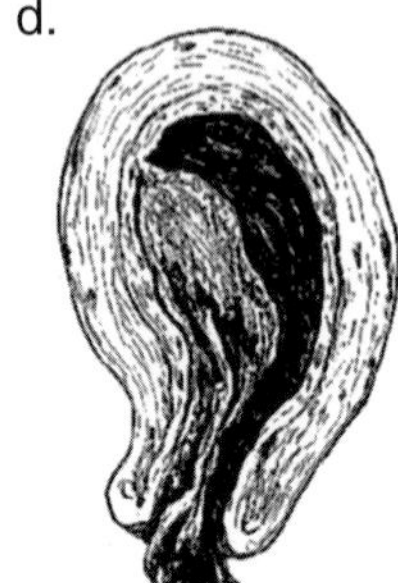

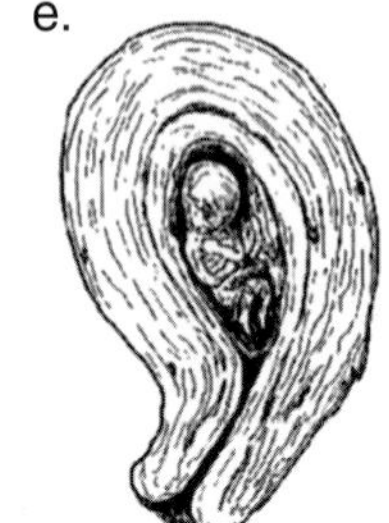

63.

a. Describe the physical findings.
b. What is the most likely diagnosis?
c. How does this lesion form?
d. What complication can occur?
e. How should this patient be managed?

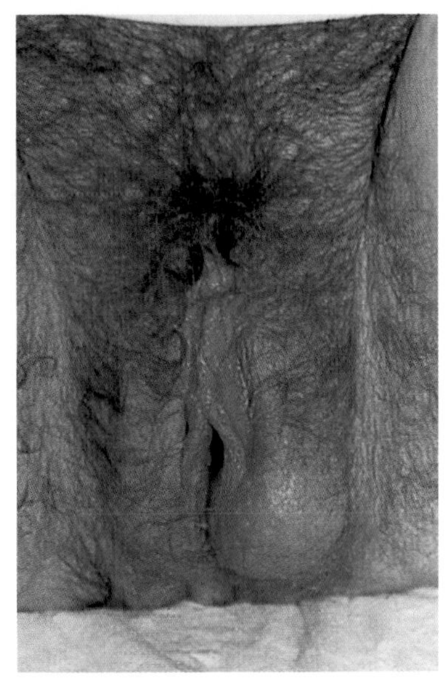

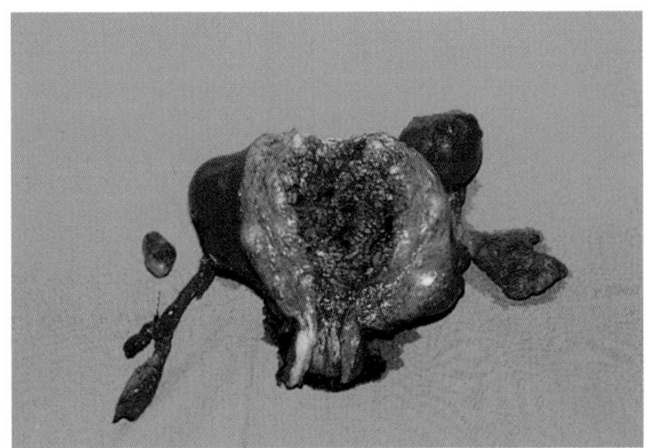

64. This woman presented with postmenopausal bleeding.

a. What is the diagnosis?
b. List the typical risk factors.
c. How is the diagnosis usually confirmed?
d. What is the typical histology of this lesion?
e. What are the characteristic patterns of spread?
f. What are the principles of management?

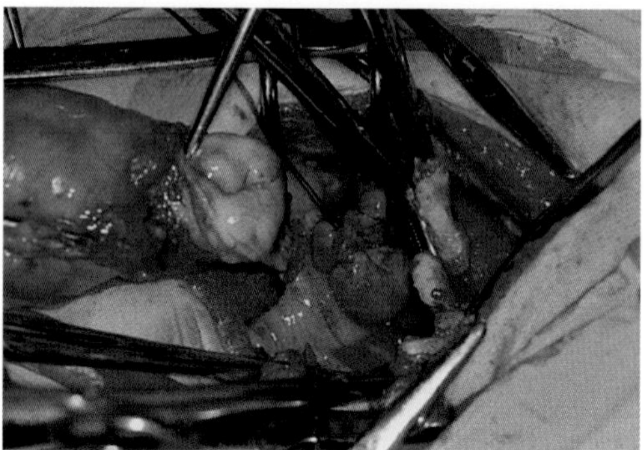

65.

a. What operation is being performed?
b. Have the ovaries been removed?
c. What structure is stained blue?
d. What suture has been used to tie the pedicles?

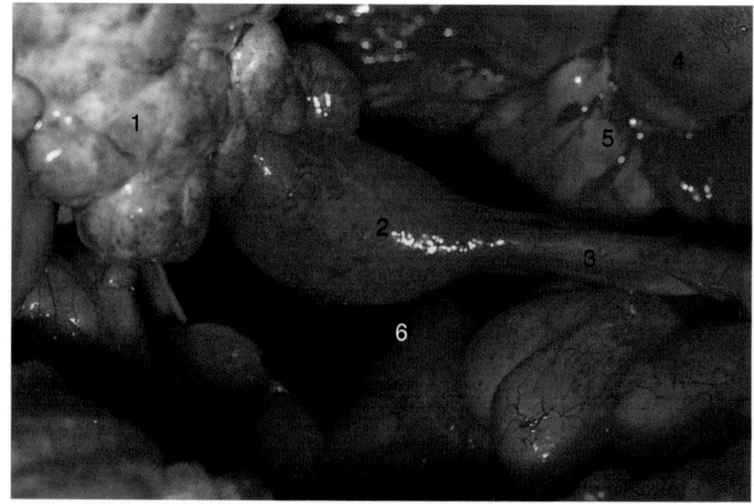

66. This woman has a left ovarian fibroma. Name the structures that are numbered 1 to 6.

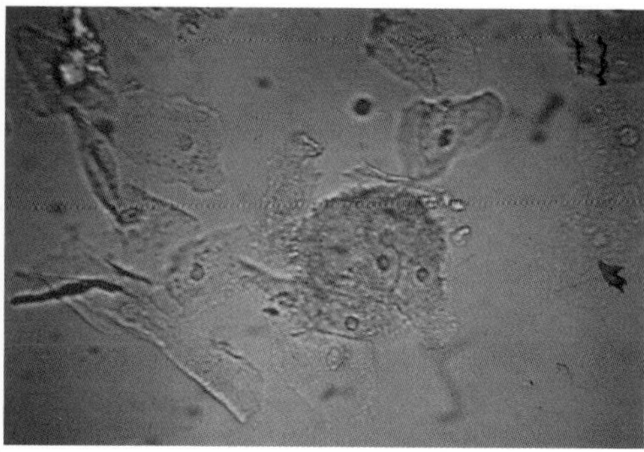

67.

a. What is the commonest cause of vaginitis?
b. What clue is present in the illustrated Gram stain?
c. What is the composition of the clue?
d. Describe the typical resultant vaginal discharge.
e. How should this vaginitis be treated?

68. These adhesions were noted between the liver and anterior parietal peritoneum.

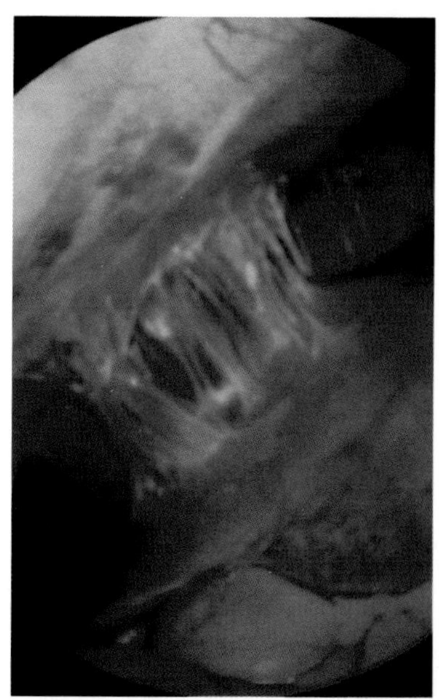

a. What is the name of this condition?
b. What is the aetiology?
c. What is the commonest infective organism?
d. How does this condition usually present in gynaecology?
e. What is the treatment?

69.

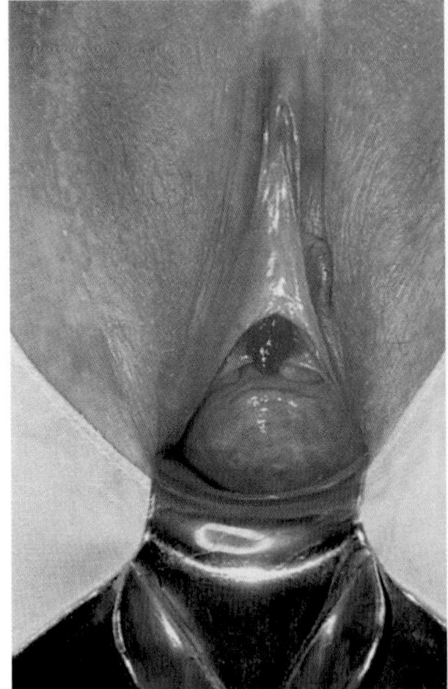

a. What is the bulging structure?
b. What structure underlies the bulging tissue?
c. With what symptoms may this patient have presented?
d. What operation will correct this abnormality?
e. What urethral abnormality is evident?

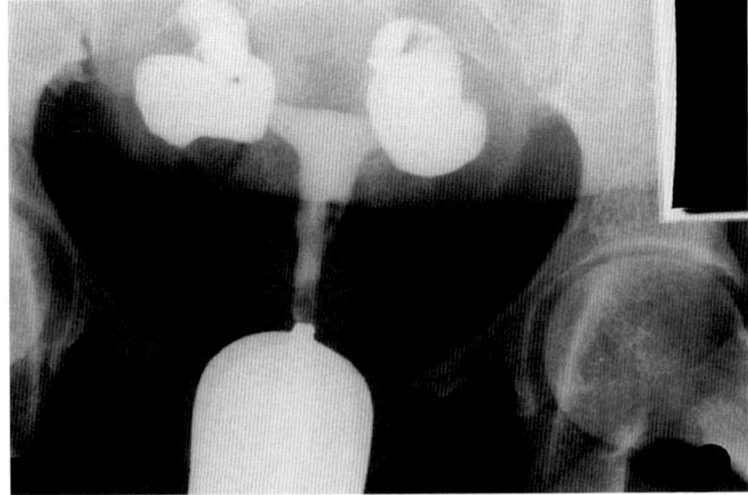

70.

a. What does this hysterosalpingogram reveal?
b. What is thc most likely cause?
c. At what level is the blockage present?
d. If infertility is the patient's main concern, what treatment options are available?

71.

a. What operation is being performed?
b. What are the supporting structures of the uterus?
c. What surrounding structures are at risk of damage during this procedure?
d. What complications can occur postoperatively?

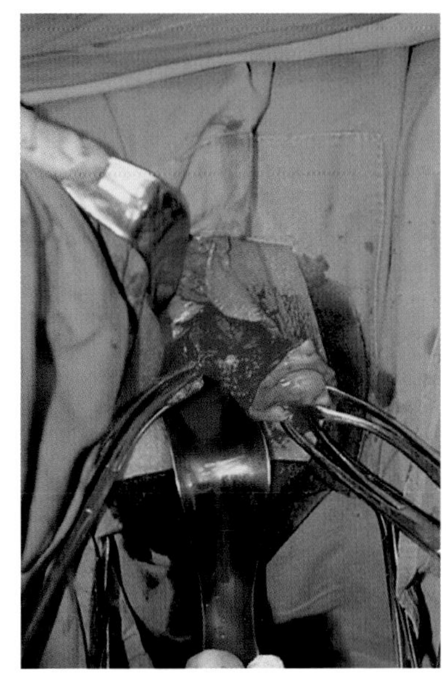

72. This lesion was present in a postmenopausal woman.

a. What is the diagnosis?
b. What is the most likely presenting symptom?
c. What is the typical histology of this lesion?
d. How would you manage this patient?
e. How would you manage this lesion in a young woman?

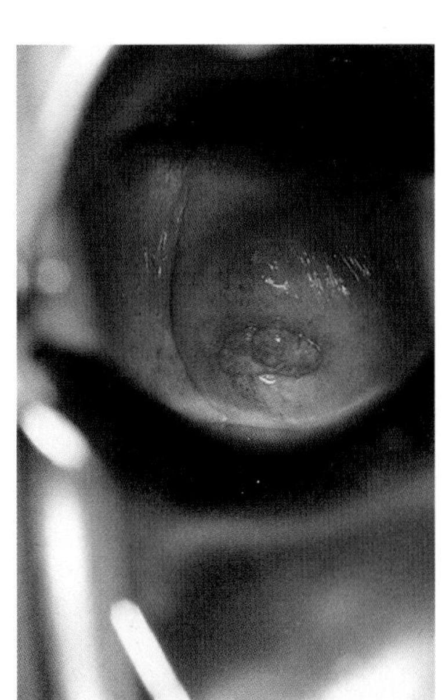

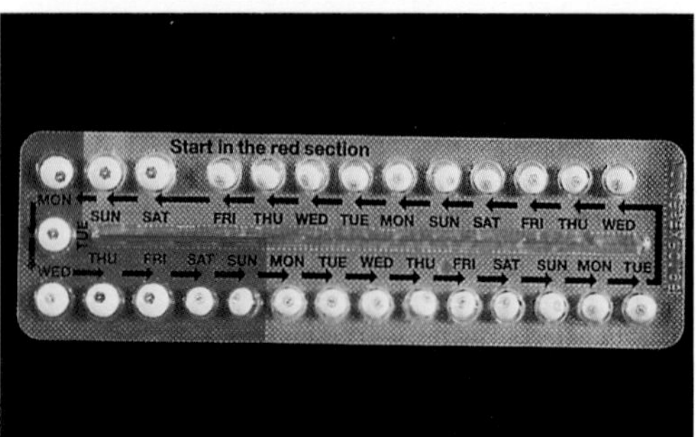

73.

a. What are these pills used for?
b. What do these pills (excluding the larger pills) contain?
c. Apart from the obvious benefit of this medication, name four other benefits.
d. If a woman missed the last two pills in the red section, what would you advise her to do?
e. Name two absolute contraindications to this preparation.

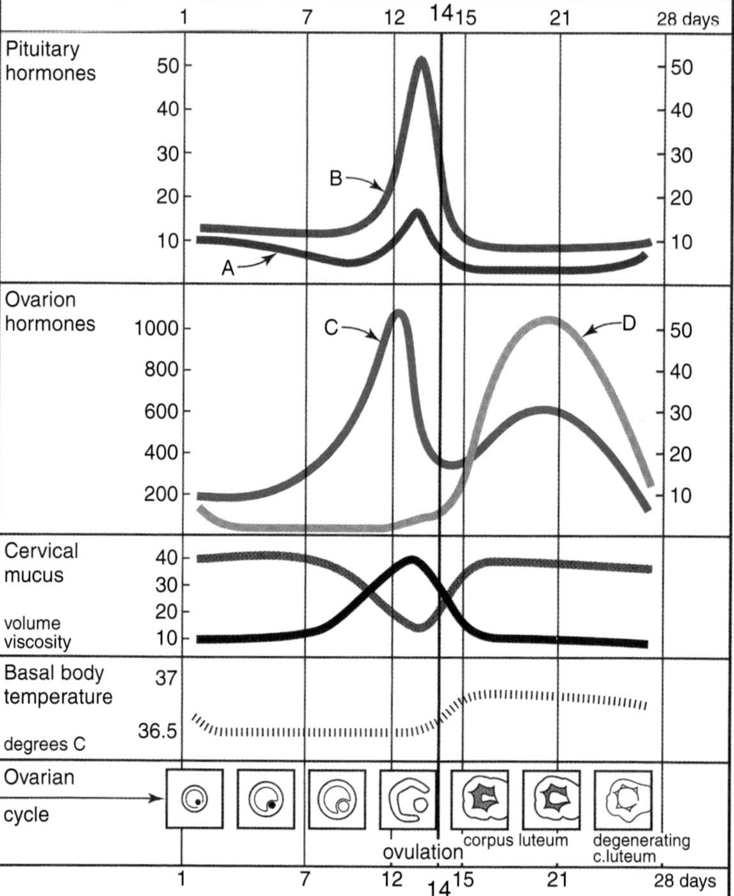

74.

a. Name the four hormones.
b. What two types of cells are involved in the synthesis of C?
c. What cells produce D?
d. What effect does D have on cervical mucus?
e. What hormone causes the temperature rise illustrated?
f. At birth, how many oocytes are present?

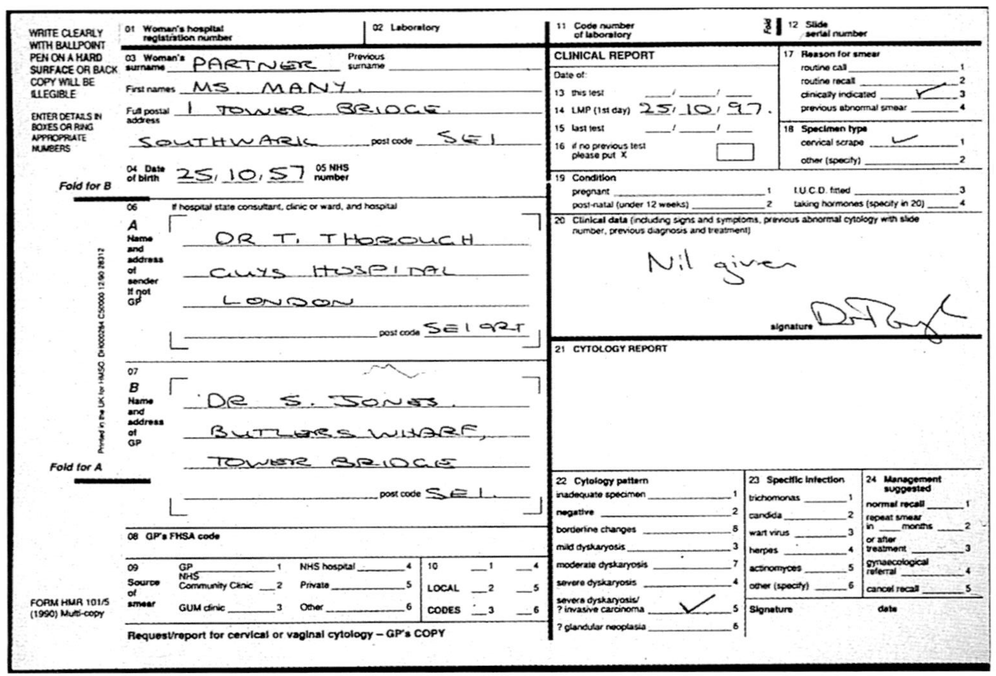

WRITE CLEARLY WITH BALLPOINT PEN ON A HARD SURFACE OR BACK COPY WILL BE ILLEGIBLE

ENTER DETAILS IN BOXES OR RING APPROPRIATE NUMBERS

01 Woman's hospital registration number | 02 Laboratory | 11 Code number of laboratory | 12 Slide serial number

03 Woman's surname PARTNER Previous surname

First names MS MANY.

Full postal address 1 TOWER BRIDGE. SOUTHWARK post code SE1

04 Date of birth 25/10/57 05 NHS number

Fold for B

06 If hospital state consultant, clinic or ward, and hospital

A Name and address of sender if not GP: DR T. THOROUGH, GUYS HOSPITAL, LONDON post code SE1 9RT

07 B Name and address of GP: DR S. JONES. BUTLERS WHARF, TOWER BRIDGE post code SE1.

Fold for A

Printed in the UK for HMSO DH000264 C50000 12/90 28312

08 GP's FHSA code

09 Source of smear: GP 1; NHS Community Clinic 2; GUM clinic 3; NHS hospital 4; Private 5; Other 6

10 LOCAL CODES 1 2 3 4 5 6

FORM HMR 101/5 (1990) Multi-copy

Request/report for cervical or vaginal cytology – GP's COPY

CLINICAL REPORT

Date of:
13 this test __/__/__
14 LMP (1st day) 25/10/97.
15 last test __/__/__
16 if no previous test please put X ☐

17 Reason for smear: routine call 1; routine recall 2; clinically indicated ✓ 3; previous abnormal smear 4

18 Specimen type: cervical scrape ✓ 1; other (specify) 2

19 Condition: pregnant 1; post-natal (under 12 weeks) 2; I.U.C.D. fitted 3; taking hormones (specify in 20) 4

20 Clinical data (including signs and symptoms, previous abnormal cytology with slide number, previous diagnosis and treatment)

Nil given

signature [signed]

21 CYTOLOGY REPORT

22 Cytology pattern: inadequate specimen 1; negative 2; borderline changes 8; mild dyskaryosis 3; moderate dyskaryosis 7; severe dyskaryosis 4; severe dyskaryosis/? invasive carcinoma ✓ 5; ? glandular neoplasia 6

23 Specific infection: trichomonas 1; candida 2; wart virus 3; herpes 4; actinomyces 5; other (specify) 6

24 Management suggested: normal recall 1; repeat smear in __ months 2; or after treatment 3; gynaecological referral 4; cancel recall 5

Signature date

75.

a. What classic symptoms may this woman have presented with? Name two.
b. As her GP, what would you do after receiving this report?
c. If the diagnosis is confirmed and is stage 1b, what is the appropriate treatment?
d. Name four risk factors for this disease.
e. What is the 5-year survival for stage 1 disease?
f. What age group has the highest incidence of this disease?

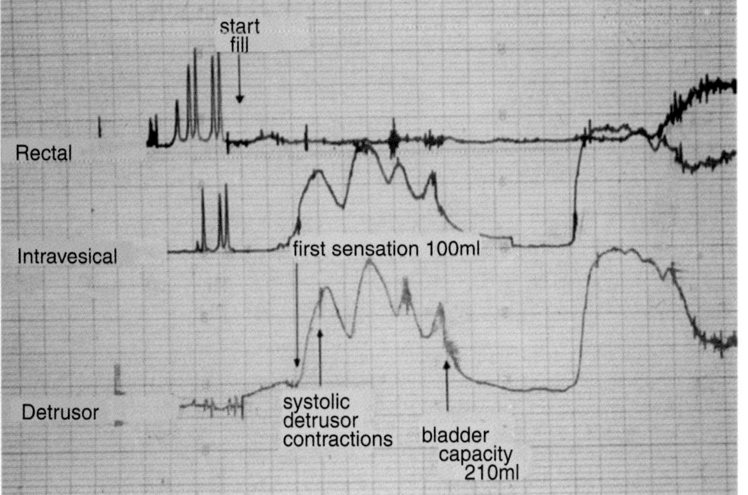

76.

a. Define urinary incontinence. Specify two features.
b. A subtraction cystometric trace is shown. Name the abnormality which is demonstrated.
c. How may a woman with this result present? Specify two symptoms.
d. What simple measures may improve symptoms? Specify two.
e. Which class of drugs may be of benefit?
f. Give an example of this class of drug (generic name with usual dose).

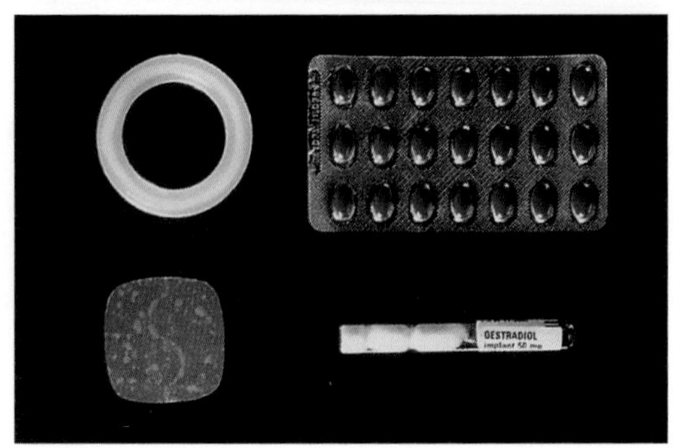

77. **The photograph shows some commonly used preparations.**

a. What is the generic term given to this group of preparations?
b. List two absolute contraindications to this treatment.
c. What are the long-term unseen benefits of such treatment? Name two.
d. In the non-hysterectomised woman, what are the alternatives to oral progestogen? Name two routes of administration.
e. What is meant by tachyphylaxis?
f. When using implants, how might you reduce tachyphylaxis?

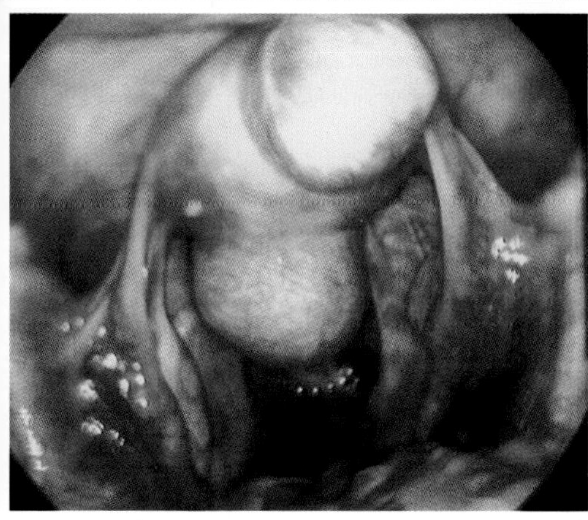

78. **This photograph was taken laparoscopically.**

a. What abnormality does it show?
b. Name three symptoms this patient may have presented with?
c. If she was to have this abnormality removed by a conservative procedure, what intraoperative complications may arise? Name two.
d. What must a patient be warned about prior to this operation?
e. If this woman had become pregnant prior to her operation, name two complications that she may have had during the pregnancy.
f. In what percentage of cases may this condition be malignant?

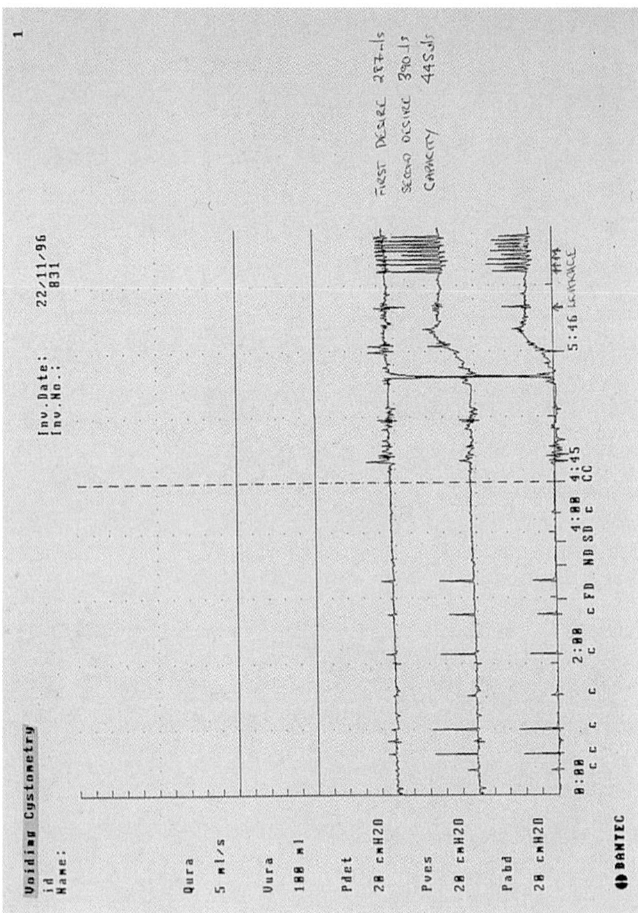

79.

a. Look at the result shown. Name the investigation.
b. Define a normal urinary flow rate for a woman.
c. What is the abnormality shown?
d. What simple measures may improve the patient's symptoms? Name two.
e. List three surgical approaches to treat this condition, and provide an example of each.
f. Which operation has the highest documented success rate?
g. What is the usually quoted success rate in experienced hands?

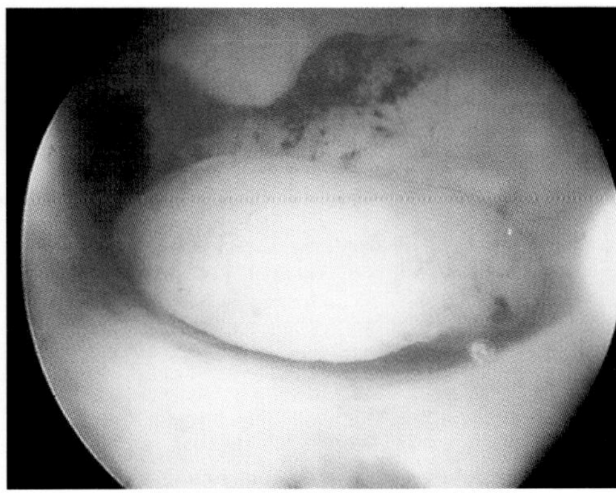

80. This woman presented with IMB.

a. What operation is being performed?
b. What can you see?
c. What management is indicated?
d. What other causes are there for IMB? Name three.
e. What media can be used to distend the cavity? Name two.
f. Is the histology likely to be benign or malignant?
g. How else might this problem have been diagnosed?

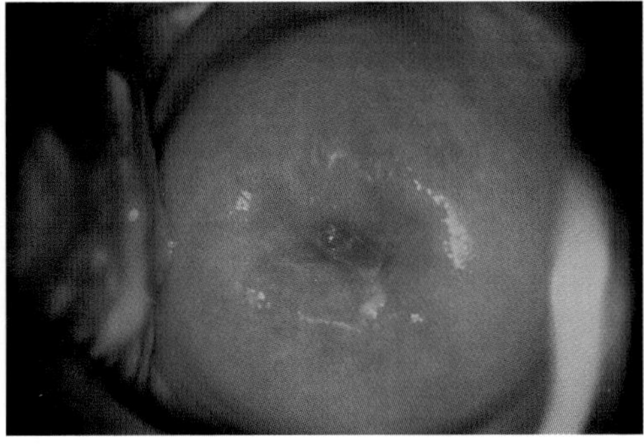

81.

a. What instrument is being used here and what does it show?
b. During this investigation what solutions are applied?
c. What is dyskaryosis?
d. What is dysplasia?

Answers

1.
a. Squamous cells.
b. Nucleus is enlarged, chromatin is increased and nuclear borders are irregular.
c. Refer for colposcopy

2.
a. Sims speculum.
b. The patient is placed in the left lateral position with the right leg bent and the left leg straight. The upper shoulder is rotated towards the bed.
c. Uterovaginal prolapse. Cases where it is difficult to visualize the cervix with Cuscoe's speculum. Suspected fistulae. In gynaecological operations. Antepartum haemorrhage.
d. Sponge forceps (to support the anterior vaginal wall).

3.
a. Intrauterine contraceptive devices.
b. Endometrial sterile inflammatory reaction that inhibits implantation. Sperm migration and ovum transport are altered.
c. Undiagnosed genital tract bleeding, pregnancy, pelvic infection, major structural abnormalities and Wilson's disease (copper devices).
d. Aseptic technique, uterus sounded, anterior lip of the cervix is grasped with a volsellum forceps and the device is inserted in the uterine cavity to the predetermined length and the strings are cut.
e. Immediate complications: pain, vasovagal shock, uterine perforation. Late complications: infection, menorrhagia, expulsion and male dyspareunia.
f. Every 5 years.

4.
a. Candidal infection (thrush).
b. Itching and vaginal discharge.
c. Microbiological swab.
d. Antifungal agents such as clotrimazole or econazole.
e. After positively confirming the diagnosis, both partners should be treated concomitantly. The female partner should be treated with a powerful oral agent such as fluconazole.

5.
a. Gram-negative intracellular diplococci.
b. Gonorrhoea.
c. Urethritis, cervicitis which may ascend into the upper genital tract, anorectal and pharyngeal infection. Septic gonococcal arthritis usually involves the knee.
d. Demonstration of the organism in culture.
e. Exclude concomitant infection, appropriate antibiotic therapy, cessation of sex during treatment, tracing of sexual contacts, follow-up for test-of-cure.

6. *a.* Female genital mutilation (FGM).
b. Difficulty with micturition, painful menstruation and dyspareunia.
c. Difficulty with cervical assessment and obstructed labour at the outlet.
d. Labioplasty – reversal of the FGM.
e. Anterior episiotomy.

7. *a.* Enlargement of the pituitary fossa and double flooring of the fossa.
b. CT, MRI.
c. Pituitary adenoma. Secondary amenorrhoea, infertility and galactorrhoea.
d. Serum prolactin, visual fields and thyroid function tests, CT of the fossa.
e. Drugs (e.g. phenothiazines, metoclopramide, methyldopa), other pituitary and hypothalamic tumours, primary hypothyroidism, pregnancy.
f. Carbergoline, hypophysectomy, and radiation therapy.

8. *a.* Cervical smear test. This is a screening test to detect abnormal cervical cells.
b. Aylesbury spatula.
c. Normal recall is 3-yearly.
d. Transformation zone.
e. The smear must be taken quickly, in the absence of blood, smeared (thinly and evenly) across a glass slide and fixed immediately.

9. *a.* Vulval carcinoma.
b. Postmenopausal women.
c. Squamous cell carcinoma.
d. Lymphatic spread to the superficial and deep inguinal and femoral nodes and then to the external iliac nodes. Direct spread occurs to vagina, urethra and anus.
e. Radical excision with en bloc dissection of the draining nodes on both sides.

10. *a.* Basal body temperature chart.
b. There is a small drop in the temperature on day 14, followed by a rise in the temperature of approximately 0.6°C that persists for 12 days. Timing of intercourse appears to have been appropriate.
c. Ovulation.
d. Day 21 progesterone (in a 28-day cycle).

11. *a.* Uterine pseudogestational sac, true gestational sac containing a fetus in the right adnexum.
b. Low abdominal pain with vaginal bleeding after amenorrhoea (classically about 6 weeks), shoulder-tip pain.
c. Unilateral abdominal tenderness, uterine size less than dates, cervical os closed, unilateral adnexal tenderness and cervical excitation, a tender adnexal mass.
d. Serial quantitative beta-HCG levels and laparoscopy.

12. *a.* Congenital tubal abnormalities, pelvic inflammatory disease, tubal surgery, intrauterine contraceptive devices, previous ectopic pregnancy and assisted conception techniques.
b. Ampulla, other portions of the tube, ovary, broad ligament, cervix and abdominal cavity.
c. Tubal abortion, pelvic haematocele, possible tubal rupture and rarely an abdominal pregnancy that progresses to term.
d. Other complications of early pregnancy, pelvic inflammatory disease, ovarian cyst accidents, bleeding from the corpus luteum and appendicitis.

13. *a.* Systemic chemotherapy, laparoscopic techniques (salpingostomy salpingectomy or injection of embryotoxic substances), open laparotomy (linear salpingostomy, segmental resection, salpingectomy). Conservative management – monitoring BHCG levels and clinical signs.
b. The original pathology is probably bilateral. Grief/bereavement counselling may be required. An early ultrasound scan is required in future pregnancies.
c. Risk is determined by the condition of the contralateral tube. Varies between 10 and 15%.

14. *a.* Carcinoma of the cervix and endometrium.
b. External beam radiation therapy, brachytherapy (source close to target), intracavitary.
c. Skin erythema and hair loss, urinary urgency and frequency, nausea and vomiting, abdominal pain, tenesmus, diarrhoea and bone marrow suppression.
d. Proctitis, rectovaginal fistula, small bowel injury with malabsorption and stricture formation, haemorrhagic cystitis, sterility and vaginal stenosis. Secondary malignancies may occasionally be seen.

15. *a.* Endometriosis. This is defined as endometrial tissue in sites other than the uterine cavity.
b. Coelomic metaplasia, retrograde menstruation and subsequent implantation, venous or lymphatic spread.
c. Symptoms are secondary dysmenorrhoea, dyspareunia, chronic pelvic pain and infertility. Signs include pelvic tenderness, ± pelvic masses or nodules, and fixed retroversion of the uterus.
d. Biopsy of the lesion.

16. *a.* The person illustrated has good breast development but no pubic hair.
b. Testicular feminization.
c. The person is a 46,XY individual with androgen insensitivity.
d. Usually after puberty with normal breast development and primary amenorrhoea.
e. Absent or scanty axillary hair, normal vulva, short blind vagina with no cervix. Absent uterus. Testes are found in either the abdomen, the groins or occasionally the labia.

17. *a.* Surgical specimen showing uterus, tubes and ovaries and an endometrial polyp.
b. No symptoms, abnormal vaginal bleeding, postmenopausal bleeding. If they protrude through the cervix they may cause dysmenorrhoea or postcoital bleeding.
c. May be detected on visual examination. At hysteroscopy they will be seen directly, and at D&C they may be felt with an instrument. An ultrasound scan may also detect them.
d. They may be removed using polyp forceps but ideally they should be resected with an operating hysteroscope. Hysterectomy is an option.

18. *a.* The primary action is to prevent ovulation, and this is supplemented by contraceptive actions at the endometrial and mucus levels and also in the fallopian tube.
b. No. There is a high level initially, which declines thereafter.
c. Failure rarely occurs.
d. Highly effective and convenient; diminished incidence of heavy bleeding, anaemia, dysmenorrhoea, premenstrual tension symptoms, endometriosis.
e. Breakthrough bleeding, delay in the return of fertility, weight gain, galactorrhoea and mild androgenic effects.

19. *a.* Colposcopy.
b. Abnormal smear, female offspring of women who ingested stilboestrol antenatally, suspicion of vaginal/vulval intraepithelial neoplasia.
c. The cervix is viewed with a bivalve speculum. Acetic acid is applied to the cervix, which is then inspected. A colposcopically directed biopsy is usually taken.
d. The need for the examination should be explained and, if there is no suspicion of invasive cancer, this should be clearly stated. An explanation of the procedure should be given in nonmedical terms. If the smear result has revealed the presence of wart virus, the sexually transmissible nature of this organism needs to be discussed. The current partner may also need to be checked, and condoms should be worn with any future new partners.

20. *a.* Fibroids.
b. Menorrhagia, dysmenorrhoea, distended abdomen, urinary frequency.
c. Gonadotrophin-releasing hormone analogues.

21. *a.* *History:* onset and duration of symptoms, pubertal and menstrual history, family history and medication intake.
Examination: weight, blood pressure, signs of virilism, hirsutism or general endocrinopathy, vaginal examination.
Investigations: serum free testosterone, other appropriate hormone assays as suggested by the history and examination, pelvic (ovarian) ultrasound and, if clinically indicated, CT scan of adrenal glands, laparoscopy.

b. An androgen-producing tumour of the right ovary.
c. Androblastomas (Sertoli cell and/or Leydig cell tumours), lipoid cell tumours, hilar cell tumours and occasionally metastatic tumours of the ovaries.
d. All signs regress apart from deepening of the voice.

22. *a.* Herpes genitalis.
b. Pain, dyspareunia, dysuria, erythema, oedema, vesicles, painful ulcers, inguinal lymphadenopathy.
c. Confirm diagnosis, admit to hospital, analgesia, catheterization if required, topical local anaesthetic, treatment of secondary infection. Aciclovir can help if commenced early. Explanation of the diagnosis and the natural history.
d. If a woman with active herpes presents in labour, delivery by caesarean section is indicated if the membranes are intact or have been ruptured for less than 4 hours.

23. *a.* Carcinoma of the cervix.
b. The mean age is 52 years. Bimodal distribution with peaks at 35–39 years and 60–64 years.
c. Intermenstrual, postcoital or postmenopausal bleeding and abnormal vaginal discharge.
d. Direct invasion into surrounding structures (vagina, uterine body, parametrium). Lymphatic and haematogenous metastasis.
e. The neck and groin nodes should be checked. Chest X-ray, intravenous pyelogram, examination under anaesthetic (cystoscopy, bimanual rectovaginal examination, cervical biopsy, D&C). Additional procedures may include a skeletal X-ray and proctoscopy.
f. *Stage 1:* carcinoma confined to the cervix.
Stage 2: spread to either the upper two-thirds of the vagina or the parametrium but without extension to the pelvic side wall.
Stage 3: involvement of the lower third of the vagina, extension to the pelvic side wall and all cases with hydronephrosis or a nonfunctioning kidney.
Stage 4: spread to adjacent structures such as bladder or rectum or spread to distant organs.

24. *a.* Cuscoe's.
b. Dorsal position.
c. The labia are parted with the left hand in order to visualize the introitus. The speculum is inserted and rotated clockwise with the blades together in a posteroinferior direction. Once the speculum is in place the blades are separated and the cervix is visualized between the blades.
d. Bimanual examination to assess the pelvic organs.

25. *a.* Benign cystic teratoma (dermoid).
b. In young females particularly between the ages of 20 and 30 years.

c. This lesion derives from the primary germ cell layers and can contain structures such as hair, epidermis, cartilage, bone and, of course, teeth. Many other structures can also be found.
d. 10%. The contralateral ovary must always be inspected.
e. Malignant germ cell tumours are rare, especially in young females.

26. *a.* Normal columnar epithelium.
b. Nabothian follicle.
c. Immature metaplasia.
d. Original squamocolumnar junction.

27. *a.* Hirsutism.
b. The Ferriman and Gallway system, in which various parts of the body are graded for the degree of hair growth.
c. Idiopathic, ovarian (polycystic ovarian syndrome, androgen-producing tumours), adrenal (Cushing's syndrome, congenital adrenal hyperplasia, androgen-secreting tumours), drugs.
d. Serum testosterone, LH, FSH, SHBG.
e. Reassurance, local treatment, bleaching agents, plucking, shaving, waxing, electrolysis, drugs (oral contraceptive pill, cyproterone acetate, spironolactone). Drug therapy must be for a minimum period of 18 months.

28. *a.* Pessaries.
b. Shelf, Hodge, ring pessary.
c. Shelf, ring pessary: uterovaginal prolapse (patient declines or is unsuitable for surgery); while awaiting surgery or in order to aid healing of decubitus ulceration; in pregnancy. Hodge pessary: this is used in order to antevert a retroverted uterus.
d. Vaginal discharge, ulceration, vaginal bleeding, discomfort, impaction if neglected.
e. 4–6-monthly.

29. *a.* Laparoscopy.
b. Carbon dioxide.
c. Any organs that are within the peritoneal cavity.
d. The bladder must be emptied and an EUA must be performed.

30. *a.* CIN III and normal squamous epithelium.
b. No.
c. Yearly smears.
d. Severe dyskaryosis.

31. *a.* Left fractured neck of femur.
b. Osteoporosis.
c. The spine, radius, neck of femur.
d. Prolonged oestrogen deficiency, steroids, hyperparathyroidism.
e. Significant morbidity and a 20% mortality in the first year.

32. *a.* Osteoporosis and vertebral crush fracture.
b. Back pain, loss of height; in some cases no symptoms.
c. Early menopause, white Caucasian, family history, past history of prolonged amenorrhoea or oligomenorrhoea.
d. Trabecular bone.
e. Anxiety about going out of doors and fear of further fractures, depression, difficulty in obtaining clothes to fit and respiratory problems if the rib cage rests on the pelvic brim.

33. *a.* Bone densitometry.
b. Mid-thirties (although this is somewhat contentious).
c. Adequate calcium intake and weightbearing exercise.
d. Less than 1% per year.
e. 1–6% per year or greater (typically 2–3%).

34. *a.* Dual energy X-ray absorptiometry.
b. Bone mass.
c. Single photon absorptiometry, dual photon absorptiometry, quantitative computer tomography, plain X-ray and ultrasound.
d. Ward's triangle is an area in the neck of femur that measures the earliest site of postmenopausal bone loss.
e. Decreased scanning time, increased precision.

35. *a.* Insertion of a hormone implant.
b. Estradiol and/or testosterone.
c. As a form of hormone replacement therapy.
d. Every 6 months.
e. If the woman has a uterus she should have progestogens.

36. *a.* Turner's syndrome.
b. 45, XO.
c. Short stature, webbed neck, increased carrying angle, sexual infantilism, primary amenorrhoea and widely spaced nipples.
d. No.
e. Ultrasound scan (cystic hygroma), chorionic villus sampling, amniocentesis, cordocentesis.

37. *a.* Hydropic vesicles.
b. Trophoblastic disease.
c. Amenorrhoea followed by vaginal bleeding. Exaggerated symptoms of pregnancy.
d. Typical signs of pregnancy. Uterine size variable but normally larger than dates. Absent fetal heart sounds.
e. Confirm diagnosis with ultrasound scan. Suction evacuation of uterus. Careful monitoring of HCG level. Registration with an appropriate centre. Advise avoidance of pregnancy for 6 months to 2 years.

38. *a.* Hysteroscopy.
b. CO_2, glycine or normal saline.
c. Visualize the endometrial cavity. Procedures can also be performed through the hysteroscope, e.g. removal of endometrial polyps or endometrial ablation.

39. *a.* Intravenous pyelogram (IVP).
b. Bilateral dilatation of the pelvicalyceal system. The right ureter is easily seen until the pelvic brim. Only the proximal portion of the left ureter can be seen. There is an extrinsic mass effect on the bladder.
c. Urinary urgency, frequency and symptoms secondary to renal tract infection.
d. Fibroid uterus, ovarian mass.

40. *a.* Acetic acid.
b. There is a clearly defined area of aceto white.
c. Minor lesion.
d. Nuclear atypia confined to the basal third of the epithelium.
e. Yes.

41. *a.* Normal.
b. 3 days abstinence from ejaculation, rapid transport to the laboratory of a specimen obtained by masturbation.
c. Aspiration of a sample of cervical mucus around the time of ovulation within 6 hours of intercourse.
d. Positive test: motile sperm in cervical mucus. This excludes cervical problem and confirms that vaginal intercourse has occurred. A negative test can be caused by many factors other than mucus hostility, for example poor timing or infection.

42. *a.* Absence of periods for 6 months in a previously menstruating woman.
b. Hypothalamus, pituitary, endocrine (thyroid, adrenal), ovary, genital outflow tract.
c. Anorexia nervosa. Hypothalamus.
d. Serum prolactin and FSH levels. Thyroid function test. Further investigations are determined by the clinical features and results of the baseline tests.

43. *a.* Surgery and radiation therapy.
b. The size and stage of the lesion, together with the age, weight and general medical condition of the woman.
c. The uterus and cervix together with a cuff of vagina, the uterosacral and cardinal ligaments. In addition there is a pelvic node dissection.
d. *Uppermost tape:* external iliac artery.
Lowermost tape: ureter.

44. *a.* Carcinoma of the cervix stage I and stage IIa in a woman who is non-obese, usually less than 65 years of age, and otherwise in reasonable health.
b. The common iliac, external and internal iliac, and obturator lymph nodes.
c. *Early:* haemorrhage, infection, fistula, venous thromboembolism. *Late:* bladder dysfunction (hypotonia) and lymphocyst formation.
d. Surgery allows conservation of the ovaries and leaves a functional vagina. The treatment is completed 'at one sitting' and the woman knows that the cancer has been 'removed'. There are fewer chronic bladder and bowel disturbances. Radiation therapy can be used in all stages of disease and in the vast majority of patients irrespective of their general medical condition. Ovarian function will not be conserved and the vagina may become stenosed. Long-term bowel and bladder disturbance due to radiation fibrosis can be seen in up to 8% of patients.

45. *a.* A spermatozoon.
b. Head, neck and tail.
c. Seminiferous tubules.
d. Follicle-stimulating hormone (FSH).
e. Production of testosterone.

46. *a.* 4 per 100 woman years.
b. The teat needs to be squeezed, and the sheath unravelled over the erect penis prior to any genital contact. Following ejaculation the still erect penis needs to be withdrawn while holding on to the base of the condom.
c. Provides effective contraception, portable, easy to use, does not require medical supervision and prevents sexually transmitted diseases.
d. Offer postcoital contraception.

47. *a.* The diathermy loop has been used to perform a large loop excision of the transformation zone.
b. Diagnosis and/or treatment of premalignant conditions of the cervix.
c. Cervical smear test, colposcopy.
d. Cryotherapy, cold coagulation, radical electrocoagulation diathermy, laser vaporization, cone biopsy (cold knife or laser), hysterectomy.
e. Haemorrhage, infection, cervical stenosis. A discharge occurs following the procedure and the patient should be advised to avoid the use of tampons and intercourse for the duration of the discharge.

48. *a.* Usually vague, non-specific symptoms, particularly of a gastrointestinal nature. Pressure symptoms such as urinary frequency may be present, together with lower abdominal discomfort and distention.
b. Signs of cachexia, lymphadenopathy, pleural effusions, breast pathology, ascites, omental cake lesion, mass arising from the pelvis (? fixity).

c. Full blood count, biochemical screen, chest X-ray, CA 125 level, ultrasound scan. Other tests sometimes required include barium enema and endoscopy.
d. At laparotomy.
e. Ovarian epithelial cell tumour (most probably malignant).

49. *a.* Condylomata acuminata.
b. Human papilloma virus.
c. This is a sexually transmitted disease.
d. Expectant, podophyllin (with great care), cryocautery, electrocautery, excision (rarely), laser ablation and interferon.
e. The sexually transmissible nature of the condition needs to be discussed. Obvious lesions can be removed but subclinical disease cannot be cured. Recurrences are possible and the partner needs assessment. Condoms should be worn with any new sexual partners. Regular cervical cytology is important.

50. *a.* Ovarian carcinoma.
b. The main method of spread is via the peritoneal cavity. Lymphatic and haematogenous spread also occur.
c. The omentum is a frequent site of metastatic disease, so its removal is essential in staging the disease. Omentectomy may reduce subsequent incidence of ascites.
d. The main prognostic factors are the patient's age together with stage of the tumour and amount of residual disease at completion of laparotomy.

51. *a.* Areas on the anterior lip of the cervix have been stained white with acetic acid. Mosaicism is seen along with abnormal vessels.
b. CIN III.
c. Either a colposcopically directed punch biopsy or loop diathermy.
d. No.

52. *a.* Milky discharge from both nipples.
b. Galactorrhoea.
c. Amenorrhoea or infertility.
d. Serum prolactin level and if this is raised an X-ray, CT or MRI of the pituitary fossa.

53. *a.* CIN III and invasive squamous cell carcinoma.
b. Assuming stage I carcinoma of the cervix, Wertheim's hysterectomy.
c. Yes.

54. *a.* Primary syphilitic chancre.
b. *Treponema pallidum.*
c. The incubation period averages 3 weeks but may range from 10–90 days.
d. Demonstration of spirochaetes by dark field microscopy.

e. Confirm the diagnosis and explain the need for compliance and follow-up. Exclude concurrent infections. Parenteral penicillin, abstinence from sex, contact tracing.

55. *a.* Vas deferens.
b. Vasectomy.
c. The nature and effect of the operation together with the potential irreversibility and small failure rate. Postoperatively, the patient must not consider himself sterile until semen analyses confirm azoospermia.
d. Scrotal haematoma, chronic scrotal discomfort, spontaneous reanastomosis of the vas with consequent failure, spermatic granulomas and development of antisperm antibodies.

56. *a.* Endometrial sampling in order to obtain a histological biopsy.
b. Nil.
c. Pregnancy, chronic cervicitis, current or recent pelvic inflammatory disease.
d. Insert vaginal speculum and clean cervix, apply single toothed forceps to the anterior lip of the cervix, sound the uterus, insert the sampler into the uterine cavity, steady the sampler's sheath while rapidly pulling back the piston, withdraw the sampler and express the tissue into an appropriate transport medium.
e. Uterine spasm or cramping, perforation.

57. *a.* Filschie sterilization clip.
b. Tubal occlusion.
c. The patient must understand the implications of the procedure. You must discuss the potential irreversibility, the failure rate, the risks and complications of the procedure, and the small risk of a minilaparotomy being required.
d. 2–3 per 1000.

58. *a.* Uterine body.
b. Uterosacral ligaments.
c. No, a small amount of free peritoneal fluid is commonly seen.
d. Large bowel.

59. *a.* Hysterosalpingogram.
b. Investigation of infertility (uterine anomalies, check tubal patency), check on tubal patency after tubal surgery and occasionally verification of tubal occlusion after a difficult sterilization procedure.
c. Anaphylactic reaction, pelvic pain (tubal spasm), reactivation of pelvic infection.
d. Bicornuate uterus with bilateral free spill of dye.

60. *a.* A chronic vulval dermatosis, a generalized pruritic condition, parasitic infection, contact dermatitis, VIN, glycosuria, psychological causes, candidiasis and trichomoniasis.

b. A combination of clinical appearance, response to topical treatments ± biopsy.
c. Topical high potency steroids. If no response consider biopsy.

61. *a.* Laparoscopy with dye instillation.
b. Investigation of infertility, check on tubal patency after tubal surgery.
c. *Laparoscopy:* general anaesthetic but allows full inspection of the pelvic organs and check on tubal patency.
Endometriosis and fine peritubal adhesions also seen.
Hysterosalpingography: outpatient procedure that outlines the uterus and internal tubal structure, but the false negative rate, due to tubal spasm, is higher. No information regarding the peritoneal cavity. The ovaries of the woman receive a dose of irradiation.
d. Normal fimbrial ends with obvious spill of dye.

62. *a.* Threatened.
b. Inevitable.
c. Complete (expelled products).
d. Incomplete.
e. Delayed.

63. *a.* Golf-ball-sized swelling in the left posterolateral vulva. No associated inflammation.
b. Bartholin's cyst.
c. These cysts result from dilatation of the duct rather than of the gland itself.
d. If infection occurs a Bartholin's abscess will result.
e. Marsupialization of the cyst is the simplest treatment.

64. *a.* Endometrial carcinoma.
b. Nulliparity, obesity, hypertension, diabetes mellitus and unopposed oestrogen therapy.
c. Hysteroscopy and endometrial biopsy or formal dilatation and curettage.
d. Adenocarcinoma.
e. Direct spread to adjacent structures, lymphatic and haematogenous spread and spillage of exfoliated cells from the tubes.
f. Total abdominal hysterectomy and bilateral salpingooophorectomy, surgical staging ± adjuvant radiation therapy.

65. *a.* Total abdominal hysterectomy.
b. No.
c. The vagina
d. An absorbable polyfilament suture e.g. vicryl.

66. 1 = left ovarian fibroma.
2 = uterus.
3 = right fallopian tube.

4 = surgeon's finger.
5 = bladder.
6 = large bowel.

67. *a.* Bacterial vaginosis.
b. A clue cell is evident.
c. The clue cell is an epithelial cell with numerous adherent bacteria. The characteristic organism is *Gardnerella vaginalis.*
d. Thin, grey, homogeneous, odorous discharge.
e. Metronidazole 400 mg orally twice a day for 5 days.

68. *a.* Fitz-Hugh–Curtis syndrome.
b. Perihepatitis.
c. *Chlamydia trachomatis.*
d. Signs and symptoms of pelvic infection and infertility.
e. Tetracycline (e.g. doxycycline 100 mg twice daily) for 14 days and ensure partner is treated.

69. *a.* Anterior vaginal wall.
b. Bladder.
c. Pelvic pressure, a feeling of something coming down, incomplete bladder emptying. Urinary stress incontinence may be present if there is rotational descent of the bladder neck.
d. Anterior colporrhaphy.
e. Urethral caruncle.

70. *a.* Bilateral hydrosalpinges with no spill of dye into the peritoneal cavity.
b. Pelvic inflammatory disease.
c. The terminal aspect of the fallopian tubes.
d. Tubal surgery (laparoscopic or open laparotomy) and in-vitro fertilization.

71. *a.* Vaginal hysterectomy.
b. Uterosacral and cardinal ligaments. Other support is provided by the uterus lying at 90° to the vaginal axis and the round and broad ligaments.
c. Bladder, rectum, urethra, ureter and small bowel.
d. Haemorrhage, infection, thromboembolic disease, sequelae of damage to surrounding structures (e.g. fistula), ileus, pelvic haematoma.

72. *a.* Cervical polyp.
b. Postmenopausal bleeding.
c. There is a stroma that contains dilated endocervical crypts. The surface epithelium is usually columnar and mucus-secreting. The surface epithelium may show squamous metaplasia.
d. Polypectomy, hysteroscopy and dilatation and curettage.
e. Twist avulsion as an outpatient procedure.

73. *a.* Contraception
b. Oestrogen and Progestogen
c. 1. Cycle control
2. Less bleeding
3. Less pain
4. Protects against ovarian cancer
5. Protects against endometrial cancer
6. Prevents bone loss
7. Alleviates symptoms of endometriosis
8. Acne Improvement
9. Protects against PID
d. Nothing
e. Active thromboembolic disease, oestrogen dependent tumours.

74. *a.* A. FSH
B. LH
C. Estradiol
D. Progesterone
b. Theca cells of the stroma and granulosa cells of the follicle
c. Luteinised granulosa cells of the corpus luteum
d. It makes mucus hostile or impenetrable to sperm
e. Progesterone
f. 2 million (1–4 million)

75. *a.* Postcoital bleeding and intermenstrual bleeding
b. Refer immediately for colposcopy and refer to gynaecologist for biopsy
c. Wertheim's hysterectomy or radiotherapy
d. 1. Large number of sexual partners
2. HPV 16 and 18
3. Smoking
4. Previous cervical intraepithelial neoplasia (CIN)
5. History of sexually transmitted disease (STD)
6. Early age of first coitus
e. 80%
f. 50–60 years

76. *a.* This is a condition in which there is involuntary loss of urine, leading to a social or personal problem with hygiene
b. Detrusor instability
c. 1. Stress incontinence/urge incontinence
2. Frequency/urgency/dysuria
3. Nocturia/enuresis
d. 1. Bladder drill/bladder training
2. Reduction in fluid intake, especially in the evening
e. Anticholinergic drugs
f. Propanthelinehydrocloride 15 mg B.D.

77. *a.* Hormone replacement therapy
b. 1. Oestrogen-dependent tumour/breast carcinoma/endometrial carcinoma
2. Active liver disease/chronic active hepatitis/acute hepatitis
c. 1. Prevention of osteoporosis/bone loss/preservation of bone
2. Prevention of colorectal cancer
d. Transdermal progestogen and intrauterine progestogen-containing device
e. Return of symptoms despite high levels of drug/oestrogen
f. Measure serum estradiol prior to administration. Strict adherence to time of giving implants (i.e. not less than 6 months apart).

78. *a.* Fibroid uterus.
b. 1. Abdominal distension
2. Infertility
3. Difficulty with micturition
4. Abdominal pain
5. Menorrhagia
c. Haemorrhage and damage to other organs, e.g. ureter, bladder, bowel.
d. A blood transfusion and/or hysterectomy may be needed.
e. 1. Abnormal lie
2. Urinary retention
3. Placental abruption/APH
f. 0.2%

79. *a.* Subtraction cystometry and uroflowmetry/urodynamic studies
b. > 15 ml/s
c. Genuine stress incontinence
d. 1. Weight loss
2. Stop smoking
3. Treat constipation
4. Pelvic floor exercises
5. Physiotherapy
6. Faradism
7. Vaginal cones
e. 1. Vaginal approach, e.g. anterior colporraphy/Pacey/Kelly repair
2. Abdominal approach, e.g. Burch colposuspension/ Marshall–Marchetti–Krantz
3. Combined abdominovaginal approach, e.g. Stamey procedure.
f. Colposuspension
g. 80–90%

80. *a.* Hysteroscopy
b. Endometrial polyp
c. Removal of the polyp
d. 1. Cervical polyp/cervical abnormality/cervical carcinoma
2. Endometrial hyperplasia
3. Endometrial carcinoma

4. Hormone therapy
5. Submucous fibroid

e. 1. Normal saline
2. Glycine
3. CO_2

f. Benign

g. Transvaginal scan

81. *a.* A colposcope. It shows a normal cervix.

b. Normal saline, acetic acid and Lugol's iodine.

c. Abnormal cells. This is a cytological diagnosis.

d. This is a histological term and describes a lesion in which part of the thickness of the epithelium is replaced by cells showing varying degrees of nuclear atypia.

Index

A

B

C

D

E

F

G

H

I

K

L

M

V

W